THYMUS ACTIVATION HEALING
胸腺活性化ヒーリング

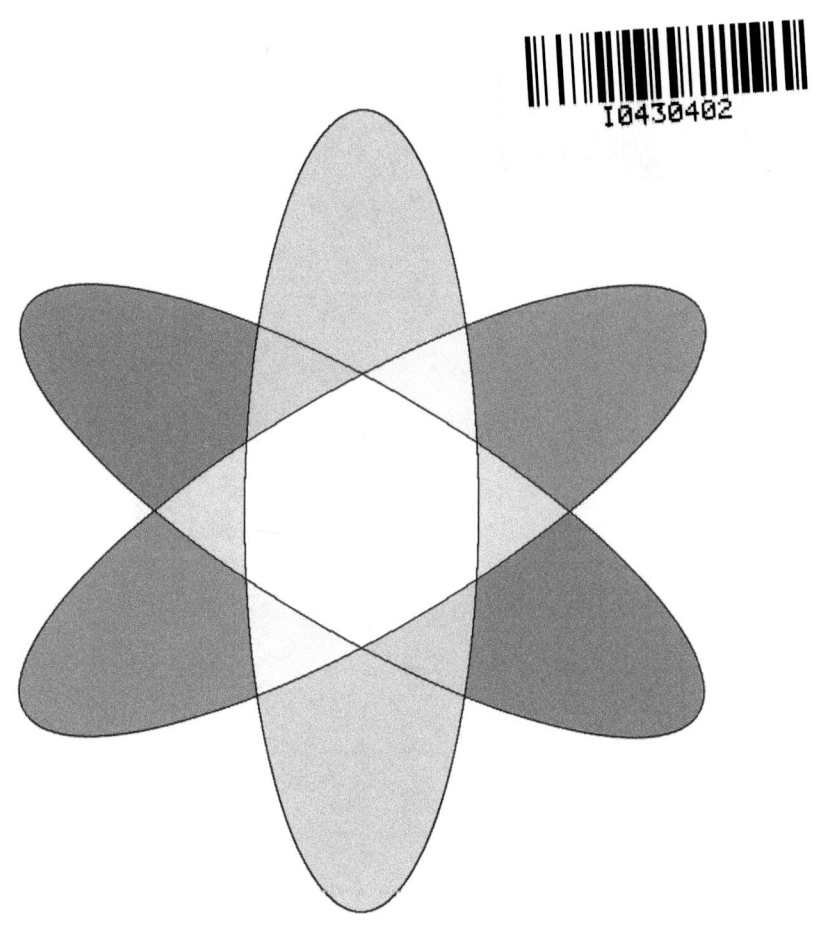

MR. TAKASHI 2BAKI
つばきたかし

Thymus activation healing
胸腺（きょうせん）活性化ヒーリング
version 1.0 revision 2

Mr. Takashi 2baki
つばきたかし

はじめに
INTRODUCTION

　Thymus activation healing 胸腺活性化ヒーリングの方法は書籍のおわりにて日本語とGoogle翻訳英語でご紹介してあります。
　The method of thymus activation healing is introduced in Japanese and Google translated English at the end of the book.

　いち早くヒーリングを試してみたい方は、お手数ですが、おわり前のページをお辿（たど）りください。
　If you want to try healing as soon as possible, please go to the end page.

それでは、はじめにヒーリングの要（かなめ）となる愛についてご紹介していきます。
First, I would like to introduce you to love, which is the cornerstone of healing.

続いて、ヒーリングを続けていった結果、何が起きたのかをご紹介します。
Next, I will introduce what happened as a result of continuing the healing.

続いて、伝授されたヒーリングと共に独自に編み出したヒーリングなどをご紹介します。
Next, I will introduce the healing that I have been taught and the healing that I have devised independently.

続いて、仮説を立てて、医学的な面からみた、胸腺の情報をご紹介します。
Next, I will make a hypothesis and introduce information about the thymus from a medical point of view.

おわりに胸腺活性化ヒーリングのやり方をご紹介します。
In conclusion, I will introduce how to perform thymus activation healing.

是非（ぜひ）、抗わずにお進みいただけたらと思います。
By all means, I hope that you will proceed without resistance.

それでは、本書をお楽しみください。
I hope you enjoy this book.

目次 TABLE OF CONTENTS

はじめに Introduction	3
目次 Table of contents	6
愛 Love	7
仙人の話 Hermit story	17
上昇気流 Ascension	29
かごめ Kagome	35
覚醒体験 Awakening experience	47
救済策 Relief policy	56
まえがき Foreword	100
本編 Main story	102
引用・参考文献一覧 Literature list	124
おまけ Bonus	128
仮説 Hypothesis	138
胸腺 Thymus	149
おわりに At the end	212

愛 LOVE

これは、愛を試したバージョンとなります。
This is the tested version of love.

愛と聞いて何を思い浮かべますでしょうか、恋愛の愛、友情の愛、親切な行動などに感じる愛などです。そういった愛が想像できるかと思います。
What do you think of when you hear the word love? The love of romance, the love of friendship, the love you feel in acts of kindness, and so on. I can imagine that kind of love.

この中に、もう一つ、真実（しんじつ）の愛を伝えるとすると、自己愛が含まれるのかと思います。
In this, I think that self-love is included if you tell one more true love.

自己愛、
Self-love

自己を愛する愛です。
It is self-loving love.

自己を愛することができれば精神的な自立が生まれます。
Self-love creates spiritual independence.

それは、どういったことかと言いますと、自分を愛するというのは、自分の体に滋養（じよう）を与えることになるんですね。そして、それと同時に、自分の体にとって愛という栄養（えいよう）を受け取ることにもなります。

In other words, loving yourself is nourishing your body. And at the same time, you receive the nourishment of love for your body.

この体にとって、これほど頼もしいことはないわけです。

for this body. It has never been so reliable.

愛を与え、愛を受け取る、そういった循環（じゅんかん）が一個人の中で芽生えてきて、愛のエネルギーのループが生まれてくると、この体は喜びに満ちた状態となって、心から嬉しく思うようになっていきます。

Giving love and receiving love, such a cycle sprouts in one individual, and when a loop of love energy is born, this body becomes a state full of joy, and you will be happy from the bottom of your heart.

これを、日常的に続けていくと、精神的な自立への道しるべとなっていって、あなた様を上昇へと導いていくことになるでしょう。

If you continue to do this on a daily basis, it will become a signpost for your spiritual independence and will lead you to an upward rise.

この上昇のことをアセンションと呼びます。

This is called ascension.

または、上昇気流と呼びます。
Or we call it an updraft.

そして、真の自己愛を体験します。
And experience true self-love.

真の自己愛に目覚めてまいりますと、他者に依存せずに生きていくことができるようになっていきます。他者からの愛を受け取らなくとも自己愛で単純に生きていける。
When you wake up to true self-love, you will be able to live without depending on others. You can live simply with self-love without receiving love from others.

と、まぁ、そういうことになるわけです。
And, well, that's what happens.

もちろん、他者からの愛も、たくさん受けて、更なる愛を享受（きょうじゅ）できるようにもなっていますから、一石二鳥といったことにもなるわけです。
Of course, we receive a lot of love from others and are able to enjoy even more love, so it's like killing two birds with one stone.

ですから、これを得（え）ない手はない。そう思います。ぜひ、あなた様の目でお確かめください。
Therefore, there is no reason not to obtain this. I think so. By all means, please check it with your own eyes.

愛の定義について
About the definition of love

　一言に愛と言っても、様々な認識があるかと思います。
　Even if you say love in one word, I think there are various perceptions.

　恋愛の愛や、友情の愛、真心のこもった親切な行動などに感じる愛などです。
　Love in romantic relationships, love in friendship, love in acts of sincerity and kindness.

　これらのことから推測できることは、愛は社会的に証明された人間生活を豊かにするための潤滑油［じゅんかつゆ］（潤滑剤やグリスやグリース）のような働きを持っています。
　What we can infer from these things is that love works like a socially proven lubricating oil (lubricant, grease) to enrich human life.

　ここでは、この働きを、エネルギー的に見る、物の見方をご提供したいと思います。それは、ハート、胸の中心、人間のセンターコア（心臓）に居る存在、自己に内在し得る存在を新しく定義させて進めさせていただきたいと思います。
　Here, I would like to offer an energetic perspective on this working of love. I would like to proceed with a new definition of the existence that exists in the heart, the center of the chest, the human center core (heart), and the existence that can be inherent in the self.

本文章の目的は、そのハートに在る、あなた自身の存在、自己に内在する存在のエネルギーの使い方を体験していただいて、愛のエネルギーの循環（じゅんかん）を体験していただきたいと思います。そして、愛のエネルギーの覚醒者になってもらえたら嬉しいです。

　The purpose of this article is for you to experience the use of the energy of your own being, the being that resides in your heart, and experience the circulation of the energy of love. And I would be happy if you could become an awakener of the energy of love.

　また、愛のエネルギーを自在にあつかえるようになってまいりますと、第一に不安を軽減することが出来る様になっていきます。もちろん、不安を完全に無くすことはできませんが、愛のエネルギーが快活されてまいりますから、下手な精神科にかかるよりも健康的ですし、不安症状からも少し、改善されて、安全で守られた健やかな効果が期待できることでしょう。

　Also, if you can handle the energy of love freely, you will be able to reduce anxiety first. Of course, you can't get rid of anxiety completely, but the energy of love will be revitalized, so it's healthier than going to a bad psychiatrist. A healthy effect can be expected.

　また、愛のエネルギーが全身を循環していくようになってまいりますと、肌の若返りや、美容効果も期待できます。

Also, when the energy of love circulates throughout the body, skin rejuvenation and beauty effects can be expected.

優しく温かい循環エネルギーに守られてまいりますから、世の中がどう混乱してこようとも、安全です。と宣言することができるようになってくると思います。

We will be protected by gentle and warm circulating energy, so I think we will be able to declare that we are safe no matter how much confusion the world may have.

また、愛のエネルギーを用（もち）いることが出来るようになってまいりますと、この世の中に存在する全ての物に対して、その物に内在するエネルギー的存在がいることを知るようになっていきます。
　Also, when you become able to use the energy of love, you will come to know that there is an energy existence inherent in all things that exist in this world.

　そうなってくると、全ての物に対して、自分と同じように内在する存在が居ることを知っていますから、自然と物を、大切に扱（あつか）っていくことができるようになっていくことでしょう。
　When that happens, you will come to be able to treat things naturally and with care, because you will know that there is an existence that is inherent in all things, just like yourself.

　そして、物をただの物として、捉（とら）えるようなことがなくなっていきますから、その物に内在する存在を愛していくことができるようになっていることでしょう。そうすると、粗末（そまつ）に物を捨てたりとか、大切に扱わないような態度は無くなってくるのではないかと思います。
　And since you will no longer perceive things as mere things, you will be able to love the existence that is inherent in those things. Then, I think that attitudes such as throwing away things poorly or not treating them with care will disappear.

また、物に内在する存在が居ることを知ってまいりますと、妄（みだ）りに人の物を欲しくなったり、盗んだり、はたまた略奪（りゃくだつ）したりといったことも少なくなってくるのではないかと思います。

Also, if you come to know that there is an existence inherent in things, I think that you will be less likely to want, steal, or loot other people's things.

　それは、その物に内在する存在が居ることを知っていますから、その存在が、その主人（持ち主）を愛していることに自然と気が付いてまいりますから、その物に内在する存在の想いが自然と伝わってきて妄（みだ）りに人の物を欲しがったり、盗んだり、はたまた略奪（りゃくだつ）したりはしなくなってくるのではないでしょうか。

It is because we know that there is an existence that is inherent in the object, and we will naturally notice that the existence loves its master (owner), so the feelings of the existence that is inherent in the object will naturally come to us.

I think that people will stop coveting, stealing, and plundering other people's things.

　これは、物に対してだけの思想ではなくて、人に対しても適用できる思想となってくると思います。それは、好きな人ができたとして、その人には別の好きな人がいて、手が出せない状況に似ているのではないかと思います。叶わぬ恋だと知ったとしても、妄（みだ）りに人の恋人を欲しがったり奪（うば）ったりはしなくなってくるのではないでしょうか。

I think that this is not just a thought for things, but a way of thinking that can be applied to people as well. I think it's similar to a situation where you can't get your hands on someone, assuming that you've found someone you like, but that person also likes someone else. Even if you know that your love will never come true, you will probably stop wanting or stealing someone else's lover.

　また、愛を用（もち）いて物事を考えれるようになってまいりますと、心を用いて物事をとらえれるようになっていきますから、その好きな人と一緒に居る、憎（にく）き相手に対しても自分と同じように愛を用いれる尊（とうと）い存在である素質を持った人だと言うことを知っていますから、妬（ねた）んだり嫉（そね）むようなことも少なくなってくるのではないでしょうか、極端（きょくたん）な話をするならば憎いからといって人を殺してしまうような無惨（むざん）な姿は無くなってくるのではないでしょうか。
　Also, when you learn to think with love, you will be able to perceive things with your heart. Therefore, I know that even the person I hate who is with the person I love is someone who has the potential to be a "precious" being who can use love in the same way as I do. Therefore, I think that envy and jealousy will decrease. To take an extreme example, I think the tragic appearance of killing people just because they hate them will disappear.

そこに愛の真骨頂（しんこっちょう）があるのではないかと思います。

I think that there is the true value of love.

また、愛のエネルギーを用（もち）いれるようになってまいりますと準備が整った段階で上昇気流（アセンション）が起こります。

Also, when you are ready to use the energy of love, an upward current (ascension) will occur.

次章より、その体験の一部をご紹介して、愛と友情のエネルギーの使い方をお伝えしてまいりたいと思います。

From the next chapter, I would like to introduce some of the experiences and tell you how to use the energy of love and friendship.

仙人の話 HERMIT STORY

　昔の仙人と呼ばれる人達が、こぞって不老不死を唱えていた理由が、もしかしたら、このことなんじゃないかって思うようなことが見えてきました。
　In the past, I began to see that this might be the reason why the people called hermits were all advocating immortality.

　この章では、このことについて書いていきます。
　I will write about this in this chapter.

　不老不死の意味はいつまでも年をとらず死なないことと言われています。
　It is said that the meaning of immortality is to never grow old and never die.

　しかし、昔の仙人たちは死んでいっています。彼らが言いたかったことは、いつまでも年を取らずに若々しく見える生き方を実現されて、それを、言葉にして表現されていたんじゃないかって思い始めているわけです。
　But the old hermits are dying. I'm starting to think that what they wanted to say was that they were able to realize a way of life that looked youthful without getting old, and that they were expressing it in words.

人間である以上、死はあるんだけど、人間に与えられている潜在的能力を使って、いつまでも若々しくいられる方法を仙人達はあみだしていたのではないかと考察しているわけです。

As long as we are human, we are bound to die, but I think that the hermits may have devised a way to stay youthful forever by using the latent abilities that humans are endowed with.

　結果的に、あの人、いつまでも死なないよねって言われる仙人と呼ばれる存在になっていったのではないかと推測を立てています。

As a result, I speculate that he became a being called a hermit who is said to never die.

　ですから、一般常識や、現代の科学のレベルでは到底理解できない何かを彼らは発見して、それを体得していた。と、そう思うわけです。が、しかし、文献に出てくる仙人の話は目にするものの、本物の仙人に僕は会ったことがないので、おとぎ話くらいにしか思っていませんでした。

So they discovered something that they couldn't understand at the level of common sense or modern science, and they were familiar with it. That's what I think. However, although I've seen stories about hermits in books, I've never met a real hermit, so I thought of them as little more than fairy tales.

しかし、天然石業界で有名なロバート・シモンズさんからクリスタルヒーリングを学び、好きこそ物の上手なれの言葉の通りに、毎日クリスタルヒーリングを続けていった結果、僕はアセンション体験をしました。日本語に訳（やく）すと上昇気流を体に感じるレベルで体感したと言うことです。

However, I learned crystal healing from Mr. Robert Simmons, who is famous in the natural stone industry. As the saying goes, if you like what you do, you are good at it. As a result of continuing crystal healing every day, I had an ascension experience. In other words, it means that I experienced the rising air current at a level that I can feel in my body.

　これにより、「目に見えない系」の世界のお話が現実味を帯びてきました。本当に人間の体には秘密がいっぱい備わっていて、科学では解明されていない未知の領域が、どうやら本当にあるようだ。と思ったわけです。

　As a result, the story of the "invisible system" world has become more realistic. The human body really has a lot of secrets, and it seems that there really is an unknown area that has not been elucidated by science.

僕も、昔は、現実主義者と言いますか、目に見えない系のお話は、敬遠するほど、見向きもしなかったタイプの人間でした。しかし、本当にアセンション体験をすると、無視なんてできないどころか自分から発信したくなる現状にあります。

In the past, I was also a realist, the type of person who didn't pay much attention to stories about invisible systems. However, when you really experience ascension, you can't ignore it, and you're in the current situation that you want to send it yourself.

これ、マジもんやん。ヤバァってことです。
This is a real story. I was really surprised.

僕の話をしますと、アセンション体験を味わうと、毎日、欠かさずアセンションをするようになっていきました。ヒーリングの仕方も、クリスタルを外したヒーリングを独自に編み出していって、愛と友情のエネルギーの使い方という方法に落とし込んで、今でもブラッシュアップしています。

As for me, once I tasted the ascension experience, I began to ascend every day without fail. As for the method of healing, I have devised a unique method of healing without crystals, and I am still brushing it up by applying it to the method of using the energy of love and friendship.

そんな中、２０２２年の５月中旬頃〜６月初旬頃にアセンション体験のクライマックスと言いますか、目覚めの体験と言いますか、恐怖体験こみの覚醒体験を経験しました。これは、非常に伝えづらい内容になるのですが、喜びと表裏一体である正反対の現象が現れ出でました。これには本当に注意が必要です。

In the midst of this, from around mid-May to early June 2022, I had the climax of my ascension experience, an awakening experience with fear. This is a very difficult content to convey, but the diametrically opposite phenomenon that is inextricably linked to joy has emerged. This requires extreme caution.

その経験の中で、僕は、ハートの中心より少し上側にある、言葉では伝えづらい場所にある存在の活性化を経験しました。

In that experience, I experienced the activation of existence in a place that is difficult to describe in words, slightly above the center of my heart.

このことから、これはなんだと、興味を持つようになっていって、図書館にある医学の本を片っ端から調べていったところ、どうやら、医学の世界では胸腺（きょうせん）と呼ばれている存在であることがわかってきました。

From this, I became interested in what this was, and when I looked up all the medical books in the library, it seems that it is what is called the thymus in the medical world. I understood that it was the thymus.

この経験から、胸腺（きょうせん）には、人間の免疫機能を司るT細胞を成熟させる器官であることがわかってきました。ガンやコロナなどの病気も胸腺さえ活性化できてしまえば、有利になる。そう言うことが言えるようになります。

　From this experience, it has become clear that the thymus is an organ that matures T cells that control human immune functions. Diseases such as cancer and corona will be advantageous if even the thymus can be activated. You will be able to say that.

　このことから、胸腺の活性化が起これば免疫機能がアップして行くわけです。そして、どうやら、覚醒体験まで進むことができれば、胸腺の存在を肌感覚で認知できるようになり、日々、愛と友情のエネルギーの使い方を実践して胸腺を活性化していくことができるようになる。と、まぁ、そう言うことが言えるようになってきています。

　From this, if the activation of the thymus occurs, the immune function will go up. And if you can progress to the awakening experience, you will be able to recognize the existence of the thymus with skin sensation. You will be able to activate the thymus by practicing the use of the energy of love and friendship every day. I'm starting to be able to say that.

一応、補足しておきますと、胸腺（きょうせん）の感覚を認知できる。と、表現しましたが、これは、特別な意味を含（ふく）みます。

I'll make a supplement. I described it as being able to perceive the sensation of the thymus. but this has a special meaning.

実際の覚醒体感の流れの中では、体が敏感（びんかん）になり過ぎて、性別をも超越したような感覚を味わい、その結果、様々な臓器が活性化されていく流れの中で、胸腺（きょうせん）の蝶（ちょう）の姿とも思えるような感覚を感知しました。

In the actual process of awakening, my body became too sensitive and I felt like I was transcending gender. As a result, in the process of activating various organs, I sensed a sensation that resembled a "butterfly" in the upper part of my chest (thymus).

僕の場合、蝶番（ちょうつがい）とも表現できるような気もしていますし、翼（つばさ）にも例えられるような気もしています。鳥のように感知される方もおられるかと思います。おそらく、人によって捉え方や感じ方が変わってくるのではないかと想像しているわけです。

In my case, I feel that it can be described as a "hinge", and I also feel that it can be likened to a wing. I think some people perceive it like a bird. Perhaps, I imagine that the way people see and feel will change depending on the person.

よって、ここに表現された以外の様々な表現方法がこれから世の中に現れ出てくると思います。僕は、そういった特別な感覚を味わいました。

Therefore, I think that various ways of expression other than those expressed here will appear in the world in the future. I had such a special feeling.

もちろん、このことを実証する必要があると思います。が、しかし、僕は医者でもなければ、医療関係者でもない。ですから、証明の仕方がわからないわけです。また、僕だけに起こった覚醒体験なのか、誰にでも起こりうる体験なのかも検証が必要になるでしょう。僕の経験で言わせていただくと、覚醒体験まで実質3年かかりますから。

　Of course, I think we need to demonstrate this. However, I am neither a doctor nor a medical practitioner. So I have no idea how to prove it. Also, it will be necessary to verify whether it is an awakening experience that happened only to me or an experience that can happen to anyone. In my experience, it takes three years to experience awakening.

　これを、検証したり臨床試験のような形で証明しようとしようものなら、その技術体系が確立するまで、いったい何年かかることでしょう。僕が生きている間に立証できるかどうかも、現時点では未知数です。
　If we try to prove this in the form of verification or clinical trials, how many years will it take until the technology system is established? Whether or not I can prove it in my lifetime is also unknown at this point.

　ですから、今この記事を読んでいる、あなたはラッキーです。
　So, now that you are reading this article, you are in luck.

もし、この記事を読んで、アセンション体験や覚醒体験をしてみたい方がいらっしゃいましたら、本書の続きを熟読ください。愛と友情のエネルギーの使い方をご紹介させていただきます。

　If you read this article and would like to have an ascension experience or an awakening experience, please read the rest of this book carefully. I would like to introduce you to how to use the energy of love and friendship.

話を元に戻しますと、昔の仙人と呼ばれる人達は、この覚醒体験を経て、胸腺の活性化を体得して、その体験を活かして生きていたのではないかと、想像しているわけです。仮説の域を出ませんが、昔の医療のレベルだった頃（５００年くらい前）に、この体験をして、活用していたら、まるで仙人のようになれていたのかなぁと僕は空想をしています。

Going back to the original story, I imagine that the ancient hermits learned the activation of the thymus through this awakening experience and lived by making the most of this experience. It's just a hypothesis, but I'm imagining that if I had this experience about 500 years ago when medical care was at the level of the past, I might have become like a hermit.

　現代は、医療のレベルが上がりすぎていて、死ねない時代とさえ言われる時代に変化してきていますから、今更、仙人にならなくとも医学の力で解決できる時代になっています。

In modern times, the level of medical care has risen too much, and it is changing to an era that is even said to be "an era in which we cannot die." Therefore, we are now in an era where we can solve problems with the power of medicine without becoming a hermit.

が、しかし、人間の自然治癒力で長生きできるんだったら、自然治癒力のチカラを用いた方が気分的にいいよね。と言い逃げして、本編の真髄をご紹介差し上げたいと存じます。

However, if you can live long with the natural healing power of human beings, it would be better to use the power of natural healing power. Then I would like to introduce the essence of the main story.

それでは、ここからは、覚醒体験当時のお話も交えながら上昇気流（アセンション）の体験談や、対応策や救済策など処世術をご紹介していきます。

From here, I would like to introduce the experience of the rising air current (ascension) and the relief policy, including the story at the time of the awakening experience.

上昇気流
ASCENSION

　上昇気流（アセンション）体験は人によって、見え方や感じ方が変わってくる可能性がございます。これからご紹介する内容は一つの例としてとらえていただけたら幸いです。これからお伝えすることが必ず起こると言うわけではないことを、あらかじめご了承いただければと思います。

　The updraft (ascension) experience may look and feel different depending on the person. I would appreciate it if you could treat the contents I will introduce from now on as "one example". Please understand in advance that what I am going to tell you about will not necessarily happen.

　僕の体験談として、お伝えしてまいります。
　I will tell you as my experience story.

　2019年7月中旬に、僕は、とあるセミナーに参加しました。そこで、クリスタルヒーリングと出会い。毎日のようにクリスタルヒーリングを続けていきました。

　In mid-July 2019, I attended a certain seminar. That's where I met Crystal Healing. Since then, I have continued to practice crystal healing on a daily basis.

３ヶ月が経った頃、初めてのアセンションが始まる前に起きたことが印象的だったのご紹介しておきます。クリスタルヒーリングをしている時に、イメージの中で、基底部と言いますか、股（また）の間の中心から大きな蓮（ハス）の花が咲き、花弁（はなびら）が開いていくイメージが見えました。

About three months later, before the first Ascensions began, I would like to share with you what struck me as something that happened. When I was doing crystal healing, I saw an image of a large lotus flower blooming from the base, or rather, from the center between the legs, and the petals opening.

　また、初めての上昇気流（アセンション）が始まった頃、まどろみの中で、ハートの中心に光り輝くお光を感得しました。それは、夢見心地の中で、ハートの中心をのぞき込んで見るようなイメージでした。

Also, when the first ascending air current (ascension) began, I felt a brilliant light in the center of my heart in my slumber. It was like looking into the center of your heart in a dreamy state.

　この頃、自己に内在する存在をハッキリと認識し、実在している感覚を肌で感じ、人体の不思議に直面していった時期だったと認識しています。

I recognize that around this time, I was able to clearly recognize the existence inherent in myself, feel the sense of reality with my skin, and face the wonder of the human body.

初めてハートに昇ってくる上昇気流（アセンション）を、体感した時は、さすがにおどろきました。
When I first experienced the rising air currents (ascension) rising into my heart, I was truly astonished.

　「なんじゃこりゃぁっ」と言った感じです。
It's like saying, "What the hell is this?"

　あの体験以降、ちまたで言われている、目に見えない系のお話や、アセンションや、波動上昇、次元上昇などのお話が、頭のおかしい特定の人達のお話ではなくて、誰にでも起こりうる事象であることを知りました。
Since that experience, stories about invisible systems, ascension, vibrational rise, and dimensional ascension that have been talked about in the streets can happen to anyone, not to specific crazy people. I know it's an event.

　また、上昇気流（アセンション）がハートの上のノドあたりに差し掛かった時の頃。
Also, when the rising air current (ascension) was approaching the throat above the heart.

　アーーーーーーーーーーーーーーーンと鳴り響（ひび）く、低い重低音、どっしりとした中域音、かすかに響（ひび）く高音、大勢の声が唱和しているかのようなサラウンドで聞こえてきて、ビックリしたことを今でも覚えています。

I was surprised to hear the sound of "Ah————n", low deep bass, solid midrange sound, faint high-pitched sound, and surround sound as if many voices were chanting together. I still remember that.

このあたりまでで、だいたいクリスタルヒーリングを始めて３ヶ月〜６ヶ月くらいの間に起こったことだったと記憶しています。
Up to this point, I remember that it happened about 3 to 6 months after I started crystal healing.

また、クリスタルヒーリングを始めて半年過ぎたあたりの頃に、クリスタルを用いなくとも愛のエネルギーを用いれるようになっています。と自己に内在する存在からのお告げがあり、それ以来、クリスタルを外した、愛と友情のエネルギーの使い方を実践していきました。
Also, about half a year after starting crystal healing, I was able to use the energy of love without using crystals. Since then, I have practiced using the energy of love and friendship without crystals.

期間で言うと、クリスタルヒーリングを半年間、愛と友情のエネルギーの使い方を２年と４ヶ月くらい実践したことになります。合計して２年と１０ヶ月です。
In terms of period, I practiced crystal healing for half a year, and practiced how to use the energy of love and friendship for about two years and four months. 2 years and 10 months in total.

上昇気流（アセンション）を続けて行く過程で、いつの頃からか、ノドより上の頭蓋（ずがい）の中まで上昇気流（アセンション）が起こるようになっていきました。

In the process of continuing the updraft (ascension), at some point, the updraft (ascension) began to occur up to the inside of the skull above the throat.

そして、２年と１０ヶ月が経った頃、
Two years and ten months later,

上昇気流（アセンション）は頭蓋（ずがい）の中の先へと移り進んで行く中で、希望の光を授（さず）けます。しかし、それは、人によっては地獄絵図ともなりましょう。僕はもがき苦しみました。

The Ascension bestows a ray of hope as it moves further into the skull. However, it can also be a picture of hell for some people. I struggled.

結果、「抗（あらが）わずに進む者が勝ち」と言う言葉を授かっていながら、抗わずにはいられなくなるような性別を超越した身体の状況に直面して、せっかく教えてもらっていた言葉があるにもかかわらず、我慢の限界を迎え、身体に起こる現象に対して、初めて抗ってしまいました。

As a result, even though I had been given the saying, "The one who advances without resistance wins," I faced a gender-transcending physical situation that made me unable to resist. Despite the language, I reached the limit of my patience, and for the first time I resisted the phenomenon that occurred in my body.

そして、寒気や悪寒や恐怖感や不安感にさいなまれ、死をも覚悟した瞬間をむかえるのでした。その詳細は秘密にさせていただきますが、まさに地獄絵図でした。
　And then, tormented by chills, fear, and anxiety, he faced a moment when he was prepared to die. I will keep the details secret, but it was truly a picture of hell.

　そして、僕は男だ。男なんだ。って言い聞かせる、おまじないを言い始めるほどに追い込まれて行き、ただひたすらに耐え忍ぶのでした。
　And I'm a man I'm a man I was driven to the point where I started saying a spell, and I just endured it.

　そして、ここから、覚醒体験へと突入して行きます。
　And from here, we will rush into the awakening experience.

かごめ KAGOME

　かごめ、かごめ、かごのなかのとりは、いついつでやる、よあけのばんに、つるとかめがすべった、うしろのしょうめんだぁ〜れ。

　Kagome, Kagome, Kago no naka no tori wa, itu itu deyaru Yoake no ban ni, turu to kame ga subetta, ushiro no syoumen daare.

　日本人なら、子供の頃、よく遊んだ歌ではあります。が、しかし、上昇気流（アセンション）体験を経（へ）て読むと、はっと、驚（おどろ）く内容に気づかされ、子供の頃、思っていたような印象の歌とは少し違うことに気が付かされました。この章では、このことについてお伝えしていきます。

　If you're Japanese, it's a song that you often played as a play song when you were a child. However, when I read it after going through an ascension experience, I was surprised by the contents of the song, and realized that it was a little different from the impression I had when I was a child. This chapter will tell you about this.

この歌は地方によって、多少、言葉が違うようです。だいたい同じことを言われていますので、この章の始めにご紹介した言葉に当てはめて表現していきます。
　This song seems to have a slightly different word depending on the region. Most of them say the same thing, so I will apply the words introduced at the beginning of this chapter to express them.

　かごめ、この言葉は、てっきり目隠しして大人数で囲む、子供の頃の遊びの歌だと、とらえていました。しかし、上昇気流（アセンション）体験を経（へ）て読むと全然そういう意味ではないことに気づかされます。
　Kagome, I definitely took this word as a childhood play song that was blindfolded and surrounded by a large number of people. However, after experiencing the updraft (ascension) and reading it, I realize that it doesn't mean that at all.

　かごめ、かごめ、このかごめは、籠（かご）の目（め）、籠目を意味しています。そうですね、三角形と逆三角形が混じり合った絵、六芒星（ろくぼうせい）の形です。
　Kagome, Kagome, this kagome means basket eyes, basket eyes. Well, it's a picture of a mixture of triangles and inverted triangles, in the shape of a six-pointed star.

　では、籠（かご）の中のとりは、どういう意味でしょう。意味は色々注釈をつけれます。一つ目は鳥居（とりい）です。鳥居とは、神社の参道入り口などに建てる門と言う意味です。

So what does "Kago no naka no tori wa" mean? The meaning can be annotated in various ways. The first is Torii. Torii means a gate built at the entrance of a shrine.

これは、僕のアセンション体験から言わせていただくと、蝶番（ちょうつがい）部分になります。医学的な部位で表現するならば人間のセンターコアでもある心臓（しんぞう）の少し上あたりに生息してある胸腺（きょうせん）です。

From my ascension experience, this is the "hinge" part. In terms of medical terms, it is the thymus that lives slightly above the heart, which is also the center core of humans.

見ようによっては鳥にも見えます。
It looks like a bird depending on how you look at it.

上昇気流（アセンション）時の体感では僕は蝶（ちょう）のように感じました。が、しかし、見方によっては鳥にも見えるかもしれません。鳥と表現しても、僕にとっては、あんまり違和感はありません。どちらにしても飛んでいくものなので。ということで、二つ目は鳥です。

I felt like a "butterfly" when I experienced the updraft (ascension). However, depending on how you look at it, it may look like a bird. Even if I express it as a bird, I don't feel any sense of incongruity. Both are flying beings. So the second is a bird.

そして、「いついつでやる、よあけのばんに、」この意味は、おそらく、いつ？いつ？その姿を表すの？夜明けの晩（ばん）だよ。と言った具合に、期待（きたい）して、まちどおしくて堪（たま）らない様子（ようす）を表（あらわ）している意味にとらえています。

And then, "itu itu deyaru Yoake no ban ni" This means, perhaps, when? When? Can you show me what it looks like? It's dawn night. I take it as meaning that it expresses the unbearable state of anticipation and confusion.

僕が初めて熱くエネルギーを帯びた蝶［ちょう］（胸腺［きょうせん］）の姿を感じた時、まさしく、夜明け前の晩（ばん）でした。

It was the night before dawn when I first felt the hot, energetic "butterfly" (thymus).

覚醒体験へと進むアセンションのクライマックスあたりで熱く滾（たぎ）る蝶（ちょう）の姿をハッキリと体感しました。

At the climax of the ascension, which leads to an awakening experience, I could clearly feel the heated "butterfly".

そして、「つるとかめがすべった、」の意味ですが、僕はこの言葉を鶴（つる）ではなく、つるっと亀が滑（すべ）ったと、とらえています。

And about the meaning of "turu to kame ga subetta," I take this word to mean that the turtle slipped smoothly, not the crane.

　絵的に説明すると、籠目（かごめ）である六芒星（ろくぼうせい）の中にある亀（かめ）の甲羅（こうら）のような絵があると思うのですが、つるっと少し回転してみてほしいです。そうすると、見えてきます。

To explain it pictorially, I think there is a picture like a tortoise shell inside a six-pointed star that is Kagome, but I would like you to rotate it slightly. Then you can see it.

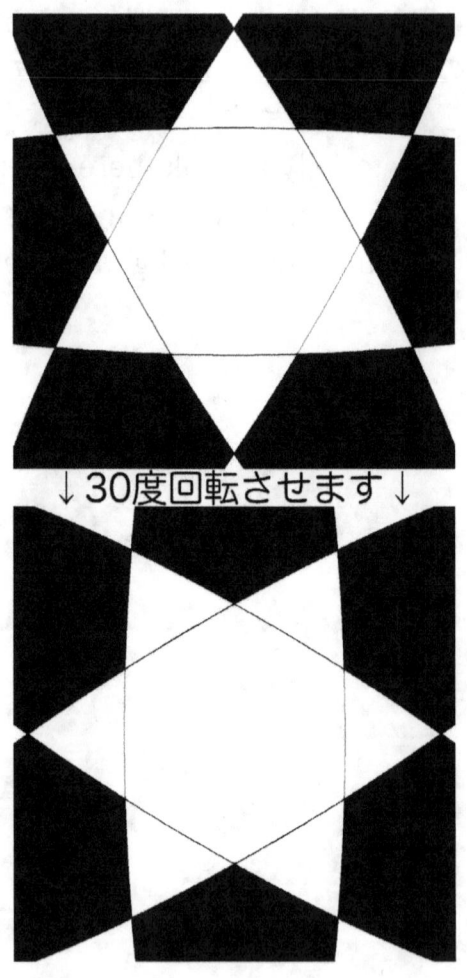

そして、「うしろのしょうめんだぁ〜れ。」これは、アセンション体験をして、目覚めと言いますか、覚醒と言いますか、「ただ、ここに、ある。」という感覚まで進まれた方でしたら、「うん」と納得できる話なのですが、なかなか一般的には理解されにくい話だと思います。

And, "ushiro no syoumen daare" This is a story that can be understood by those who have experienced the ascension experience and the awakening experience, but I think it is quite difficult to understand generally.

これは、籠目（かごめ）の鳥居［とりい］（入口）が胸腺（きょうせん）だと表現するならば、籠目（かごめ）の本殿（ほんでん）や拝殿（はいでん）は、頭のてっぺんの先、そうですね、言葉で言うには忍（しの）び難（がた）いですが。閻魔（えんま）の位置や、王冠（おうかん）の位置や、豆（まめ）の位置とも表現できます。

If the torii (entrance) of Kagome is expressed as the thymus, then the main hall (worship hall) of Kagome is the top of the head. Well, it's hard to put into words. It can also be expressed as the position of Enma, the position of the crown, or the position of the beans.

個人的な見解で言うならば、「うしろのしょうめんだぁ〜れ。」は、具体的に示すと、自己に内在する存在のことだと僕は見ています。

From my personal point of view, I see "ushiro no syoumen daare" as the existence that is inherent in oneself.

かごめの説明 Description of Kagome

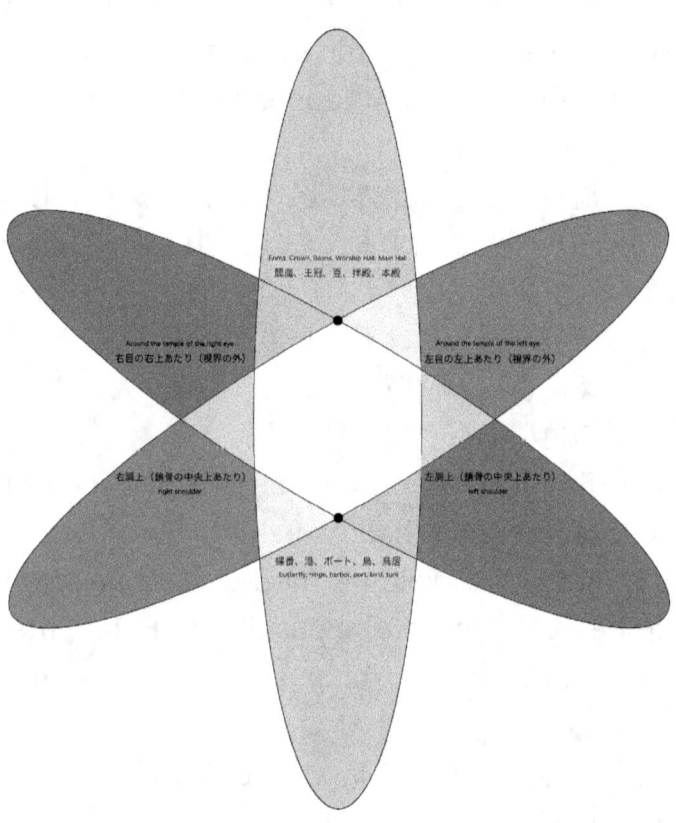

また、閻魔（えんま）と聞くと、何か怖い存在を思い浮かべるかもしれません。

Also, when you hear the word Enma, you may think of something scary.

ドラゴンボールや西遊記などのお話の影響もあって、まぁ、そのようにも、とらえられるのですが、アセンション体験をして覚醒体験をした人間にとっては閻魔は少し違った印象に映（うつ）ります。

There is also the influence of stories such as Dragon Ball and Journey to the West, and that is how it is perceived, but for people who have experienced ascension and awakening, Enma looks a little different.

閻魔とは、みめうるわしい、度を超して一つのことに熱心な人と言う意味です。少しでも閻魔の印象が変わってくれれば御（おん）の字です。

Enma means a beautiful person who is extremely enthusiastic about one thing. I would be happy if the impression of Enma changed even a little.

また、王冠（おうかん）は、頭蓋骨（ずがいこつ）の頭頂骨（とうちょうこつ）と頭頂骨をつなぐ矢状縫合（しじょうほうごう）された円状の広範囲な部分を言います。アセンション体験して行った先に現れ出でます。

Also, the crown refers to the circular wide part of the sagittal suture that connects the parietal bones to the parietal bones. It will appear after continuing the ascension experience.

また、豆（まめ）は、上昇気流（アセンション）を続けていった先に、地獄の苦しみが現れます。その地獄の苦しみを、苦しみ抜いた先に現れ出でます。

Also, the suffering of hell will appear ahead of continuing the upward current (ascension). Beans will appear at the end of that hellish suffering.

言葉では、まったく説明がつかないため、医学的な表現で説明すると、頭蓋骨（ずがいこつ）にある前頭骨（ぜんとうこつ）と左右の頭頂骨（とうちょうこつ）との間にある縫合（ほうごう）を冠状縫合（かんじょうほうごう）と言い。

Words cannot explain it at all, so to explain it in medical terms, the suture between the frontal bone in the skull and the left and right parietal bones is called the coronal suture.

その冠状縫合（かんじょうほうごう）と矢状縫合（しじょうほうごう）が交わるポイントを豆（まめ）の位置と表現させて進めさせていただきます。

The point where the coronal suture and sagittal suture intersect will be referred to as the bean position.

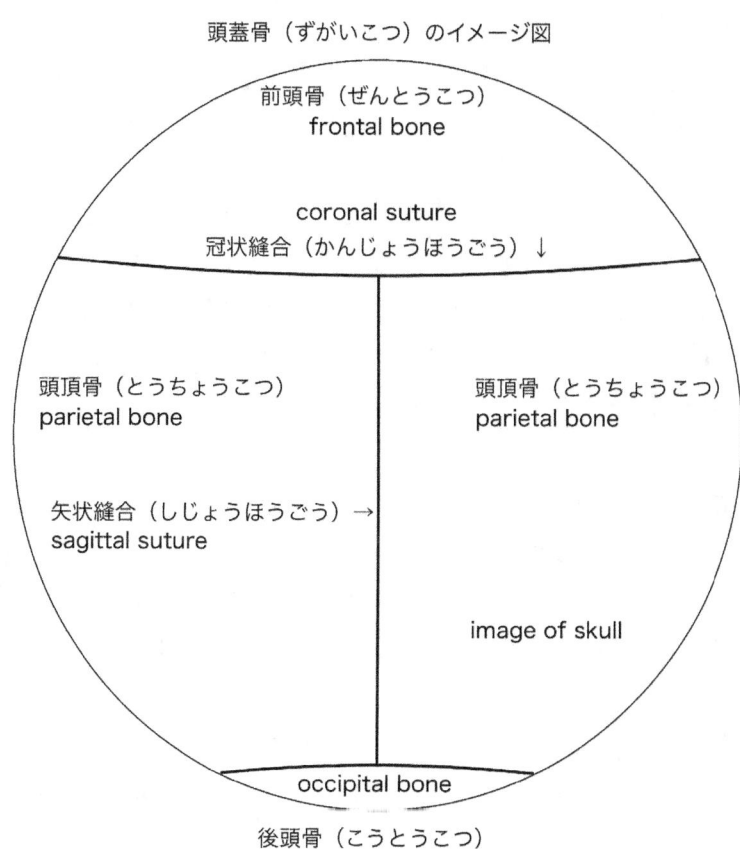

上手く伝わっていれば幸いです。
I would appreciate it if you could convey it

しかし、昔の人は良く言ったもんだなぁと感心させられます。子供の頃にその歌を歌わせて遊ばせておいて、しっかり教育されている。
However, I am impressed that the old people said well. When I was a child, I was made to sing and play with that song, and I was educated properly.

しかも、遊びの意味と内的探求の意味が上手く合わさっていて、二つの意味を成すなんて、素晴らしすぎる。
Moreover, the meaning of play and the meaning of inner exploration are well combined, and it is too wonderful to have two meanings.

まさにアセンションそのものを封じ込めていて、だれが考えたのか知るよしもありませんが、上手すぎる。
It exactly contains the rising air (ascension) itself, and I don't know who thought of it, but it's good.

歌を作った人は天才だと思いました。
I thought the person who wrote the song was a genius.

それでは、次章より、アセンション体験を進めていった先に、起こり狂う、覚醒体験した当時のお話をご紹介します。
Then, from the next chapter, I will introduce the story of the time when I had a crazy awakening experience after proceeding with the ascension experience.

覚醒体験
AWAKENING EXPERIENCE

愛と友情。そのエネルギーの使い方を知ると、上昇気流（アセンション）が起きるようになります。

love and friendship. When you know how to use that energy, the updraft (ascension) will come to happen.

上昇気流（アセンション）を使いこなせるようになると、臍下（へそした）あたりの上昇気流（アセンション）から、胸（ハート）に昇る龍となる上昇気流（アセンション）へと進化していき、喉（のど）へと昇華して、頭の中心、そして頭のてっぺんへと移り進む過程にて、スーパーアセンションとなり、地獄の苦しみと引き換えに豆を持つ様（よう）となるのです。これには注意が必要となり、身がかえるのです。

When you can master the ascending air current, it evolves from the ascending air current around the navel to the ascending air current that rises to the chest (heart) and rises to the throat and then to the head. It becomes a pattern that moves to the top of the head, and in the process of moving to the top of the head, it becomes a "super ascension", and it becomes like holding a bean in exchange for hellish suffering. This requires caution and self-recovery.

こうなってくると上昇気流（アセンション）させようと思う気持ちはなくなっていきます。それよりも、心（ハート）と頭（マァーラ）のバランスを取ろうと必死にもがきます。それが、冷や水浴びせられた模様（もよう）となるのです。

When this happens, the desire to ascend will disappear. Rather, it struggles desperately to balance the heart and the head (maala). That is the pattern of being showered with cold water.

結果的に、何もかもを手放していく姿となり、想像力すらも手放す姿となります。そして、内的探求で得た知識をも全（すべ）て覆（おお）い隠（かく）すようになります。

As a result, I seem to let go of everything, even my imagination. It also begins to obscure all the knowledge it has gained in its inner search.

ただいま、その状態にあります。
I am in that state right now.

今、僕がやっていることを明示
I'll show you what I'm doing now

　過去も未来も夢なんだ。
　空想も妄想も夢と一緒（いっしょ）なんだ。
　記憶すらも夢なんだ。
　そのことに気が付けたなら、今すぐに言ってほしい、
　目に見えるものを追いかけます。
　目に見えるものはリアルである。
　目に見えるものは今の現実なのである。
　ですから、目に見えないものを追いかけ始めたら今すぐに言ってほしい。目に見えるものを追いかけます。と、そうすれば、あなたの目（まなこ）がパッチリになって後遺症もなんのその。

　The past and the future are all dreams.
　Fantasies and delusions are the same as dreams.
　Even memories are dreams.
　If you notice that, say it out loud right now.
　Focus on the visible world.
　The visible world is real.
　The visible world is the present reality.
　So, when you start chasing the invisible world, I want you to say it out loud right now.
　Focus on the visible world. And if you do that, your eyes will be bright and there will be no aftereffects.

　これで、頭は現在に同期を始める。
　Now your head starts syncing to the present.

次にしてほしいことがあって、次って言ってもほぼ同時なんですけど、体の胴体（どうたい）と頭をつなげて同期をはかってほしいです。呼吸を実況中継してみてください。何秒吐いて、何秒吸ってとか考えなくていいです、今吐いている。今吸っている。くらいの程度でいいです。実況中継を始めると、現在に同期した頭と体の胴体（どうたい）が連動し始めます。ここに、ゆとりが生まれる様（さま）があります。

　There is something I want you to do next. Try to follow your breathing. You don't have to think about how many seconds to exhale and how many seconds to inhale. I'm exhaling air now. I'm getting air now When you start the live commentary, the head and body synchronized with the present will start to work together. There is a state that a space of the heart is born here.

　とまぁ、こう言う状態となると、気が楽になります。もし、あなたが、上昇気流（アセンション）をあつかえるようになった後、手のつけられない混迷状態になったら、この文章を読んでほしいです。きっと思考と身体がリセットされることでしょう。

　And, well, when it comes to this state, it makes me feel better. If you find yourself in a state of uncontrollable confusion after mastering Ascension, please read this article. Your mind and body will surely be reset.

この文章を書いた後、起きたことを原文のまま記述
I will explain what happened after I wrote this sentence.

　何もかも手放していき、想像力すらも手放した結果、体の準備が整ったのか、一斉（いっせい）に体の感覚すらも手放した状態となった。

　As a result of letting go of everything, and even letting go of imagination, perhaps the preparations for the body were complete, and all at once they were in a state of letting go of even the sensations of their bodies.

　それは、秘密の秘法って言われていて皆が通る道なのです。

　It's called the secret formula and it's the way everyone goes.

　自分の意思とは関係なく起こりました。そして、息もしているかどうかわからない、体の感覚すらもなくなっていて、ただ、そこに、ある。ただ、ここに、ある。と言った感覚のみとなるのでした。

　It happened against my will. And I don't even know if I'm breathing or not, I can't even feel my body, it's just there. But here it is. It was only the feeling of saying.

　思考すら存在しない感覚です。

　It is a feeling that even thoughts do not exist.

そして、頭がピクッ、ピクッっとなったかと思うと、体の感覚が戻ってきて、浅い呼吸を感じ、思考が戻ってきました。

Then, when I thought my head was twitching, the sense of my body returned, I felt shallow breathing, and my thoughts returned.

これは、いったい？…と分析を始める自分がいて、結局のところ、これまでの体験記憶から、この体験に似ている言葉を探すんだけれども、いろんな言葉が思いつき、当てはめていっても、当てはめた途端（とたん）、その言葉が嘘（うそ）に感じる感覚となり、言葉で説明することの矛盾（むじゅん）に気が付き、名前を付けると嘘（うそ）になると思うように至（いた）りました。

What is this? … Ultimately, I search for words that are similar to this experience from my past experience memories, but even if I come up with various words and try to apply them, the moment I apply them, the words has become a sense of lying. I noticed the contradiction of explaining in words. I came to think that naming it would be a lie.

無意識に瞑想（めいそう）に没入した感じ…やっぱ言葉にすると嘘（うそ）になる。笑。

I feel like I'm subconsciously immersed in meditation…, Putting it into words would be a lie.

一応、念のために、初心忘れるべからずと言う意味も込めて、僕が、その時、何を思ったのかだけ列挙しておきます。

For the time being, just to be sure, I will list only what I thought at that time, with the meaning of not forgetting my original intention.

　平安を味わう感じかな…、人様の言う無がこれか？、三昧（サマディ）がこれか？、しかし、無も三昧（ざんまい）も僕には偽（いつわ）りの言葉に見えて仕方ない。無と書くと、ただ、ここに、ある。と言う感覚があるため無ではないと結論づけれるし、三昧と書くと、心を一つのものに集中させて安定した精神状態になるさまと言う意味らしいのだが、僕自身、心を一つのものに集中させている感覚は、まったくない。自分の意思とは関係なく勝手にその状態が行われていくさまであるから、おそらく三昧（ざんまい）でもない。

　It's a feeling of peace…, Is this what you mean by "nothing"? Is this Samadhi? However, I can't help but see nothingness and samadhi as false words. If you write "nothing", you can conclude that it is not "nothing" because it has the feeling of "it is just here." It seems that the word samadhi means to focus one's mind on one thing and achieve a stable state of mind, but I myself do not feel that my mind is focused on one thing at all. This state of affairs occurs arbitrarily regardless of one's will, so it is probably not samadhi.

じゃぁ、これは、なに？と分析を進めた結果論として、この状態に名前などあるはずがないと、エクスタシーの究極点と表現してもいいが、なにか伝えている言葉の印象が変わってしまっていることに気付く。初めてこの文章を読む人に語弊（ごへい）を与えかねない。その部分だけを見ると偽（いつわ）りにも見える。また、至福（しふく）か？と分析すると、この上ない幸福（心が満ち足りていること）と言う意味らしいが…いや、そう言うことじゃないんだよなぁ…結果的にそう言う状態になるのかもしれないけれど、体感的、感覚的にはそんな印象ではなくて…。

　Well, what is this, as a result of the analysis, I conclude that this state cannot have a name. It can be described as the ultimate in ecstasy, but you notice that the impression of the words you are conveying has changed. It may be misleading to those who read this sentence for the first time. If you look only at that part, it looks fake. Also, if you analyze whether it is bliss, it seems that it means supreme happiness (satisfaction of the heart)…, No, that's not what I mean…, As a result, it may be in such a state, but it is not such an impression physically and emotionally…

　言葉にするとやはり偽（いつわ）りとなる。嘘（うそ）になる。言葉で表現できない境地とも言えるが、結局それはなんですか？となると説明つかない。

　Putting it into words would be a lie. It can be said that it is a state that cannot be expressed in words, but what is it in the end? If you ask me, I can't explain.

そう言う感覚を味わいました。
I felt that way.

そういった経験を経て思うことがあります。
I have some thoughts from those experiences.

「そうか、思考すること、そのものが夢だったんだ。」でした。
"Well, thinking itself was a dream."

もし、この文章を読んで上昇気流（アセンション）に興味を持ち、体験してみたいと思われた方がいらっしゃいましたら、愛と友情のエネルギーの使い方を体験してみてください。
If you are interested in the updraft (ascension) after reading this text and want to experience it, please experience how to use the energy of love and friendship.

これが、あなたの為（ため）となるか、どうかは、あなた自身の思考にかかっています。是非、お楽しみいただければと思います。
Whether or not this works for you is up to you. We hope you enjoy it.

救済策 RELIEF POLICY

　アセンションと呼ばれる上昇気流を堪能（たんのう）し始めると、ヘソ下あたりの上昇気流（アセンション）から、ハートあたりの上昇気流（アセンション）、ノドあたりの上昇気流（アセンション）、頭蓋（ずがい）の中へと入っていく上昇気流（アセンション）を経験していくようになります。そうなってくると、それまでの快楽や幸福感を得る楽しみとは正反対の苦楽を味わうようになっていきます。

　When you begin to enjoy the updraft called the Ascension, you will experience the updraft below the belly button (Ascension), the updraft in the heart (Ascension), the updraft in the throat (Ascension), and the updraft in the skull (Ascension). When that happens, you will begin to experience the joys and sorrows that are the exact opposite of the joys and happiness that you used to have.

上昇気流（アセンション）すればするほど、苦しみ、寒気、悪寒（おかん）を味わうようになり、ヒーリングを辞めてしまう程の、精神的に追い詰められた状態、そうですね、医学的には統合失調症（とうごうしっちょうしょう）やうつ病と診断される類（たぐ）いの症状が現れ始めます。

The more you do ascension, the more you suffer. You get chills. It will be in a mentally cornered state to quit healing. Well, you start having the kind of symptoms that are medically diagnosed as schizophrenia or depression.

　ですから、注意が必要です。
So be careful.

　僕の場合、たまたま読書が好きで、読んだ本に助けられることになりました。その結果を自分の言葉で、ご紹介したいと思います。
In my case, I just happened to like reading, and the books I read helped me. I would like to introduce the results in my own words.

過去や未来について思い悩む状態をマインドワンダリングと呼ぶ。
The state of worrying about the past and the future is called mind wandering.

　上昇気流（アセンション）が頭蓋（ずがい）の中まで入っていく上昇気流（アセンション）を体験して行った結果、寒気や悪寒、恐怖感や不安感に襲われて、精神的に追い詰められた状態に陥（おちい）って行きました。その結果、目に見えないものを追い求め過ぎている自覚が芽生え、目に見えるものを追い求めるように意識を変えて普段の生活を過ごすようになりました。
　As a result of experiencing the ascending air currents (ascension) entering into the skull, I was attacked by chills, fear and anxiety, and fell into a mentally cornered state. As a result, I became aware that I was pursuing the invisible world too much, and changed my consciousness to pursue the visible world and started to spend my normal life.

　そんな中、気が付いたことを記述します。
　In the meantime, I will write what I noticed.

今の今まで、過去の記憶が断片的にイメージで現れると、そのことについて永遠と思い出して、あの時こうだったとか、思いを巡らしていました。そういった繰り返し、ループって、実は、目に見えないものを追い求めている姿だったんだ。と気がつくようになり、あっ、目に見えるものを追いかける姿に戻ります。って宣言して戻ってみると、今の今まで、これに苦しめられていたんだって発見があり、過去の記憶って、記憶データであって、そのデータをイメージで膨らませた空想、言い換えるならば妄想なんだって気付きを得たわけです。

　Up until now, when my memories of the past appeared fragmentary in the form of images, I would remember them forever and ponder what it was like at that time. Such a repetition, a loop, was actually a form of pursuing an invisible world. I've come to realize that. I return to chasing the visible world. After declaring this, I returned and discovered that I had been tormented by this until now. I realized that memories of the past are memorized data, and fantasies inflated with images, in other words, delusions.

　それが、わかると、例えば、宝くじなんかの一等が当選したら、何しようとかいう想像、言い換えるならば妄想も、目に見えないものを追い求め過ぎている姿なんだな。と気付きがあり、そっか、これも、こうあったらいいなっていう未来予想図でしかなくて、結局のところは、過去の記憶の空想や妄想と一緒で、目に見えないものを追い求め過ぎている姿なんだな。って気付きがありました。

If you understand that, for example, if you win the first prize in the lottery, your imagination, in other words, your delusion, is a form of excessive pursuit of things you can't see. I had a realization. Well, this too was nothing more than a vision of the future that I hoped would be like this. It's proof that you're chasing too much of what you can't see. I had a realization.

正直に言うと、これもかよって気持ちにはなりましたが、目に見えるものを追い求めるように意識を変えて過ごすだけで、かなり意識改革ができるもんなんだな。と思うようになっています。

To be honest, this made me feel better. However, just by changing your consciousness to pursue what you can see, you can change your consciousness considerably. I'm starting to think.

とにかく、今は、目に見えないもの（過去や未来）を追い求め始めたら、目に見えるものを追い求める姿に戻りますと言って。リセットする癖（くせ）をつけていけたらいいな。と思っています。

In any case, I think it would be great if I could get into the habit of resetting by saying that once I start pursuing the invisible (the past and the future), I will return to the consciousness of pursuing the visible world.

しかし、目に見えるものを追い求める姿に戻っても解決できないような、寒気、悪寒、恐怖感、不安感に陥（おちい）ってしまった場合のためにも、知っておいてほしいことがあります。

But just in case you find yourself falling into chills, fears, and insecurities that returning to the pursuit of the visible just can't resolve, here's what you need to know.

それが、これ。
It is this.

薬指の秘密。リラックス法。体を脱力させる方法です。
The secret of the ring finger. relaxation method. It's a way to unwind.

手にある五本の指には、おのおの使い方や意味が存在しています。そのことを引用しながらご紹介していきます。
Each of the five fingers on the hand has its own usage and meaning. I will introduce it while quoting it.

柳生心眼流（やぎゅうしんがんりゅう）
■手の指の話、手には筋繊維として三つの流れがある。
一つ目は、親指の流れ、
二つ目は、人差し指と中指の流れ、
三つ目は、薬指と小指の流れ。
〜それそれの指の意味〜
・親指：強い力、親指は最後に頼りなさい。
（力を伝えたい時だけ使うイメージ）
・人差し指：伸ばす力
・中指：回転の指、中指を中心にして回すと手は回りやすくなる。
・薬指：交感神経、副交感神経が通っているのは薬指だけ。敏感（びんかん）。一番感覚が鋭（するど）い。
・小指：子供は家を纏（まと）める：鎹（かすがい）：小指で握ったらまとまる。

Yagyu Shinganryu

■ Talking about the fingers of the hand, there are three streams of muscle fibers in the hand.
The first is the flow of the thumb,
The second is the flow of the index finger and middle finger,
The third is the flow of the ring finger and little finger.

〜The meaning of each finger〜

・Thumb: strong power, the thumb is the last to rely on. (Use only when you want to convey power)

・Index finger: power to extend

・Middle finger: Spinning finger. Rotate around your middle finger. Hands are easier to turn.

・Ring finger: Only the ring finger has sympathetic and parasympathetic nerves. sensitive. The most sensitive.

・Little finger: Ability to gather together: When you hold it with your little finger, it will come together.

引用元：武術格闘家 菊野克紀 の 誰ツヨDOJOy
https://www.youtube.com/watch?v=8H6LtISZ8Bw

僕は、格闘家ではないため、人を殴ることは無いですが、指の意味や、指の使い方に興味があって、どんなことにでも転用できそうな気がしたので、自分なりに研究を始めています。その中で、少し、わかってきたことをご紹介しておきます。

I'm not a martial artist, so I don't hit people, but I was interested in the meaning of fingers and how to use them. I felt that it could be used for anything, so I started researching on my own. I will introduce what I have learned in it.

格闘技などの殴ることを前提とした場合、小指と薬指を握り込む形になるのかなと思います。

If you are assuming that you will hit, such as martial arts, I think it will be a form of holding the little finger and the ring finger.

殴ることに重きを置いた形 A form that assumes hitting

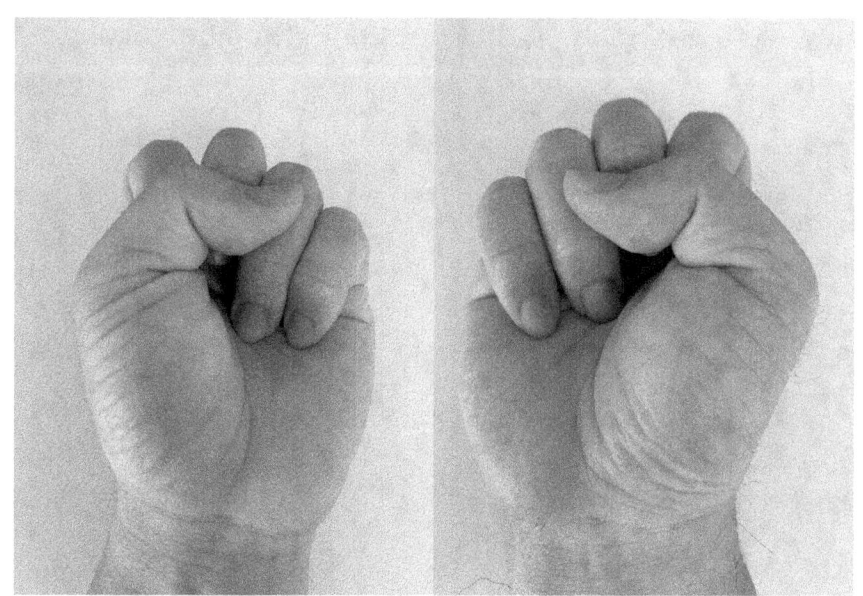

しかし、これでは、小指、薬指にどうしても力（ちから）が入ってしまうため、ウォーキングで試してみると、楽にはなるのですが、ちょっと肩の力（りき）みが発生してしまう気がして、改良を重ねていった結果、握り込まない握り方を編み出しました。ウォーキング専用です。

　However, with this, the little finger and the ring finger inevitably put a lot of force, so when I tried walking, it became easier, but I felt that the shoulder was a little strained, so I continued to improve it. As a result, I devised a grip method that does not grip. For walking only.

握り込まないグー form that does not grip

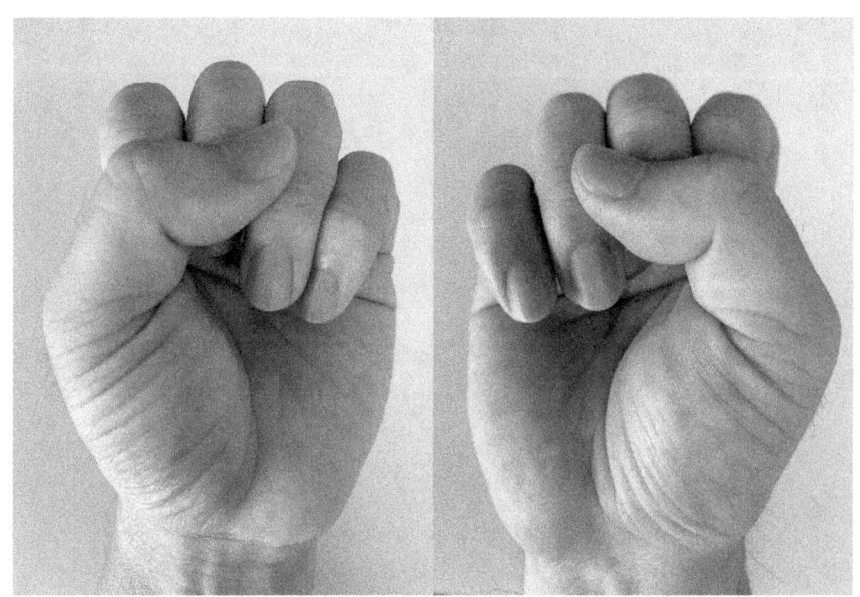

重要になるのが、親指を薬指に軽く触れるような感覚で、軽く添えるようなイメージで、握（にぎ）り込まないように、力（りき）まないようにすることが重要です。

　The important thing is to feel the thumb lightly touch the ring finger, and to have an image of lightly attaching it, and not to force it so as not to grip it.

それでは、次に、普通の人が普通に役立つ薬指の使い方をご紹介します。それは、薬指の爪に親指の腹を軽く触れるように置きます。力（ちから）は入れずにそのままの状態で過ごします。すると、肩の力は抜けていき、足の指先までぐぃーっと伸びていく感覚を味わい、今まで感じたことないような良好な感覚を味わいます。

　Next, I will introduce how to use the ring finger, which is usually useful for ordinary people. It puts the pad of the thumb on the nail of the ring finger so that it touches lightly. Leave it as it is with no effort. Then, the tension in your shoulders will go away, and you will feel the sensation of stretching all the way down to your toes.

　その効果は覿面（てきめん）です。
　The effect is great.

発見当初の形 original form of discovery

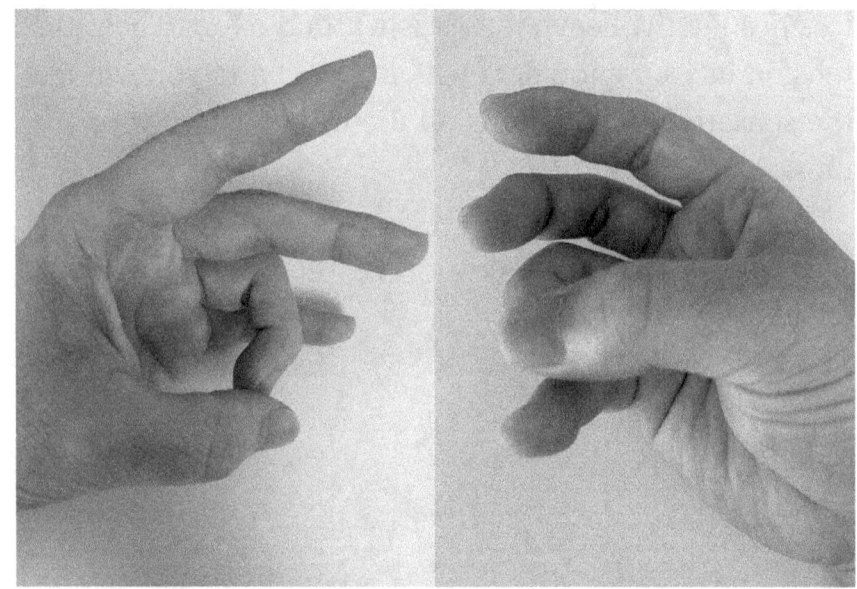

なれてくるとこうなりました。が、しかし、足の指先までぐぃーっと伸びるような感覚は減少して行きます。

This is what happened when I got used to it. However, the sensation of stretching all the way to your toes will diminish.

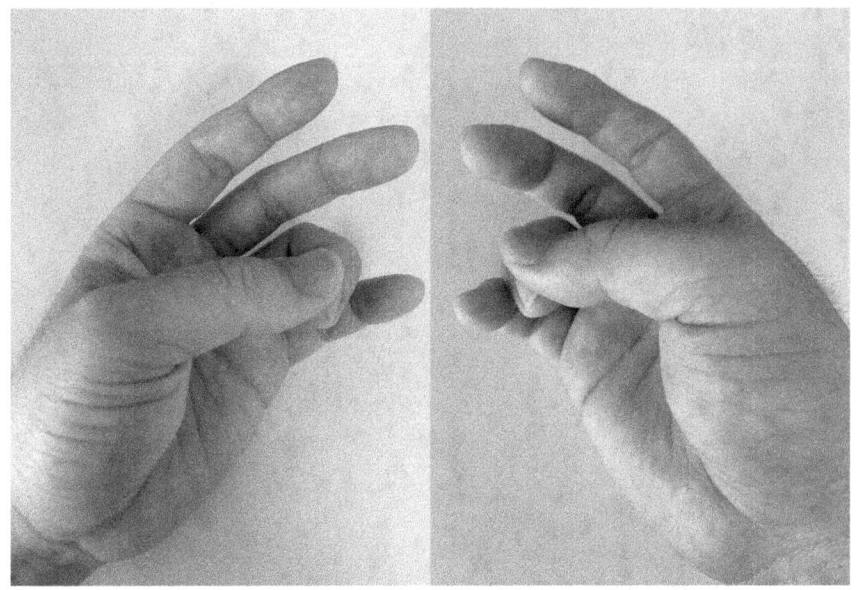

爪に当てずに指の腹同士にすると、反対のことが起こるような気がします。手がジンジンして、手が震えてくる感じ、興奮状態になっている気がします。注意が必要です。

　I feel that the opposite phenomenon occurs when I put the pads of my fingers together instead of putting them on my nails. I feel like my hands are tingling, my hands are trembling, and I feel like I'm in a state of excitement. You should be careful.

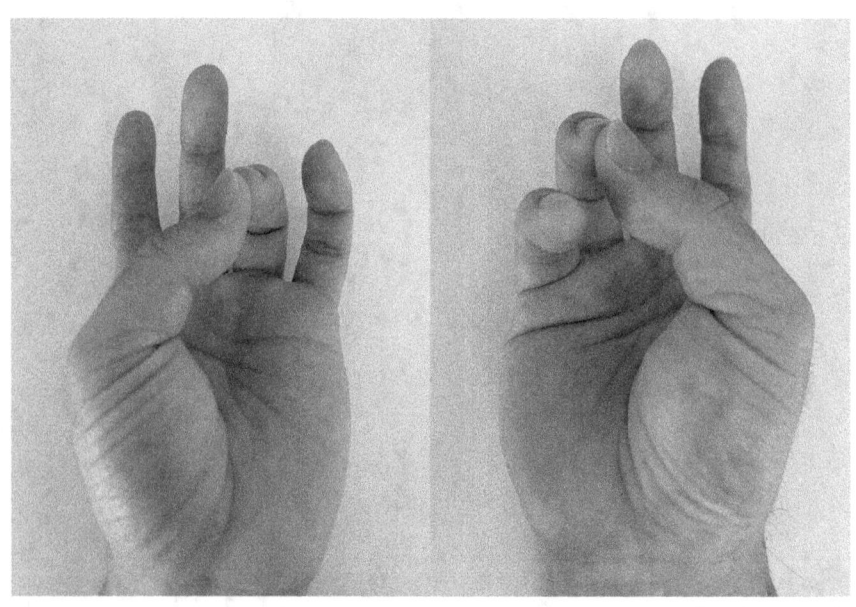

薬指の爪と皮膚に親指を触れるように添えると自然とピースになります。肩と首あたりまで守られているような感覚になりました。

If you put your thumb on the nail and skin of your ring finger, it will naturally become a piece. I felt like my shoulders and neck were being protected.

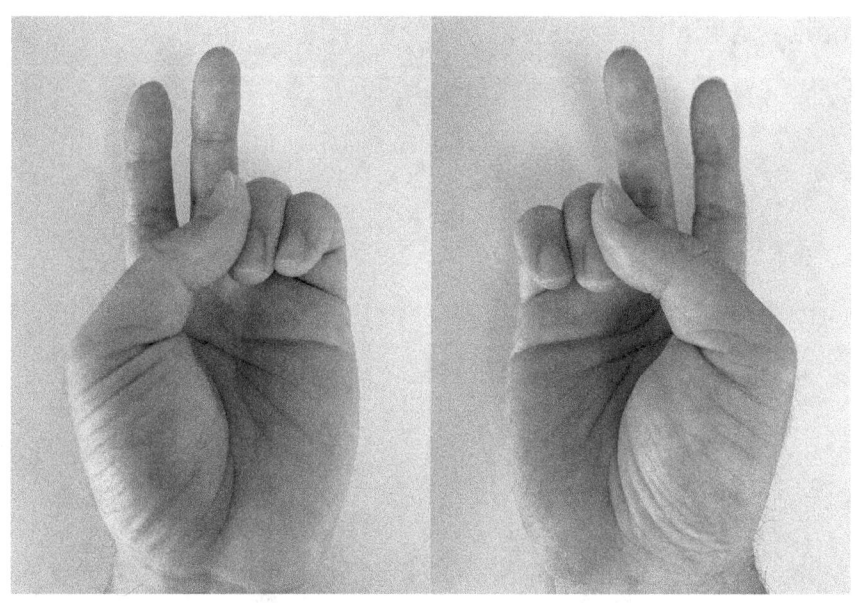

薬指の第一関節に親指の腹の先を軽く当て、親指が薬指の関節を触っている感覚がある状態を作ります。そして、親指の腹を薬指の爪に触れるように軽く置きます。本当に些細な違いですが、感覚的に大きな違いが生まれます。

Lightly touch the first joint of the ring finger with the tip of the pad of the thumb to create a state in which the thumb touches the joint of the ring finger. Then, lightly place the pad of your thumb so that it touches the nail of your ring finger. It's a really small difference, but it makes a big difference.

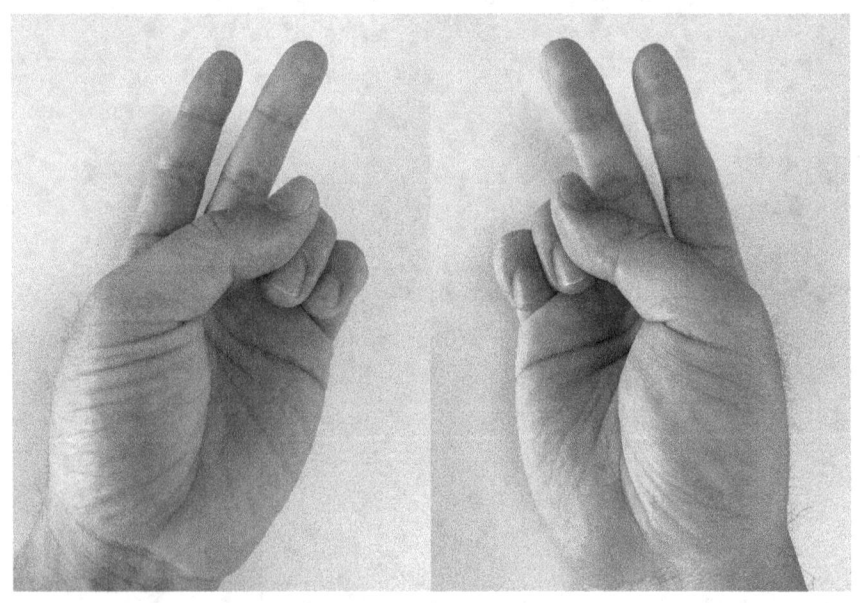

これ、スゴイって感動しています。
I'm so impressed with this.

　薬指の甲側（こうがわ）に親指の腹（はら）で触れると、全身の力が抜けていき、心まで安定していくような気がしました。副交感神経が優位の状態になっているのではないかと仮説を立てています。また、恐らくですが、薬指の手のひら側に親指の腹（はら）を置くと交感神経が優位の状態に働くのではないかと仮説を立てています。
When I touched the back of my ring finger with the pad of my thumb, I felt my whole body relax and even my mind became stable. I'm hypothesizing that the parasympathetic nervous system is in a dominant state. Also, perhaps, I hypothesize that the sympathetic nerves will work in a dominant state when the pad of the thumb is placed on the palm side of the ring finger.

　結果がすぐに欲しい場合、この形が有効だと思います。
If you want immediate results, I think this form is effective.

あと、もう一つ、ご紹介しておきます。
I would like to introduce one more thing.

　それは、薬指だけ、ほんの少し曲げる方法です。これだけです。これだけですが、意外に効果がある。効果覿面（こうかてきめん）とまではいかなくとも、ゆる～く結果が出るタイプです。普段の何気無い仕草の中に取り入れるといいんだろうな。と思っています。

　It's just a way to bend your ring finger just a little bit. Only this. This alone is surprisingly effective. It's a type that produces results slowly, even if it's not effective. It would be nice to incorporate it into the usual casual gestures.

ナチュラルにリラックスします。 Relax naturally.

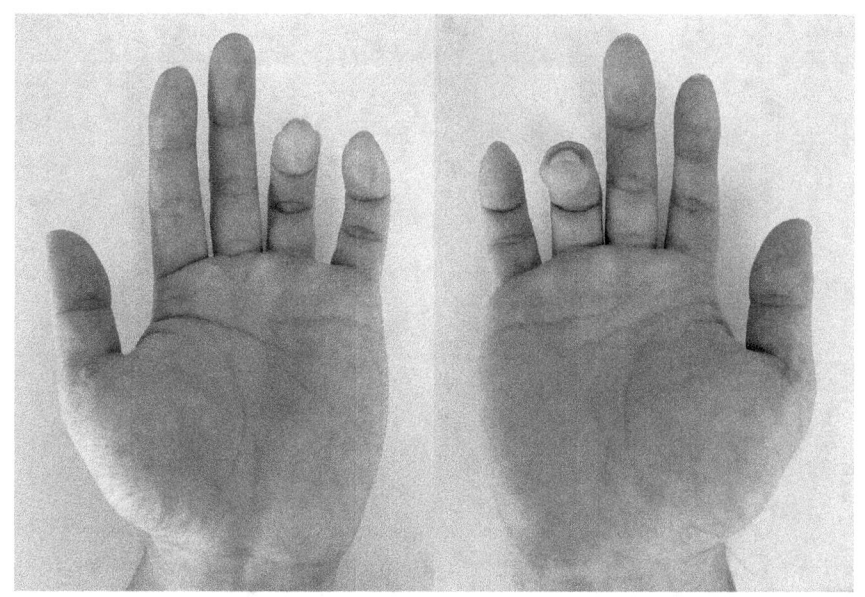

これが、薬指の秘密。リラックス法。体を脱力させる方法です。本当に困った時に思い出してみてください。

　This is the secret of the ring finger. relaxation method. It's a way to unwind. Please try to remember when you are really in trouble.

そんな中でも、教えの享受（きょうじゅ）は行われていきました。籠目（かごめ）の話や、閻魔（えんま）の話、膨大な情報量の啓示（けいじ）を受け、あまりの恐怖にメモを読む気さえ起こらない苦しみ、不安、恐怖を体験して、今でもそのメモを読もうとは思えません。

Even so, the teaching continued. The story of Kagome, the story of Enma, and the revelation of a huge amount of information, I experienced the pain, anxiety, and fear that I didn't even feel like reading my notes because I was so scared. I don't feel like reading the memo.

閻魔（えんま）の意味
Meaning of Enma

見目麗（みめうるわ）しい、王冠（おうかん）、王妃（おうひ）、生命の実を授けられた者がたどる軌跡（きせき）。えんま、漢字にすると妙（みょう）に恐ろしくなりますが、本当の意味は、閻魔（みめうるわしい、度を越して一つのことに熱心な人）と言う意味となります。

Beautiful to look at. Crown. Queen. The trajectory followed by those who are bestowed with the fruit of life. Enma is strangely scary when written in kanji, but its true meaning is Enma (a beautiful person who is extremely enthusiastic about one thing).

そう言った意味も加味してお読み頂ければ幸いです。
I would appreciate it if you could read it with the meaning of what I said.

籠目（かごめ）の意味
Meaning of Kagome

　籠目（かごめ）、文字にすると籠（かご）の目となります、平たく言うと六芒星（ろくぼうせい）です。三角形と逆三角形が交差した絵図柄（えずがら）を意味します。簡略的に伝えると光の図です。

　Kagome, when written, it becomes the eyes of a basket. It means a picture pattern in which a triangle and an inverted triangle intersect. In simple terms, it is a diagram of light.

籠目（かごめ）と呼ばれる六芒星をクローズアップ。
A close-up of a six-pointed star called Kagome.

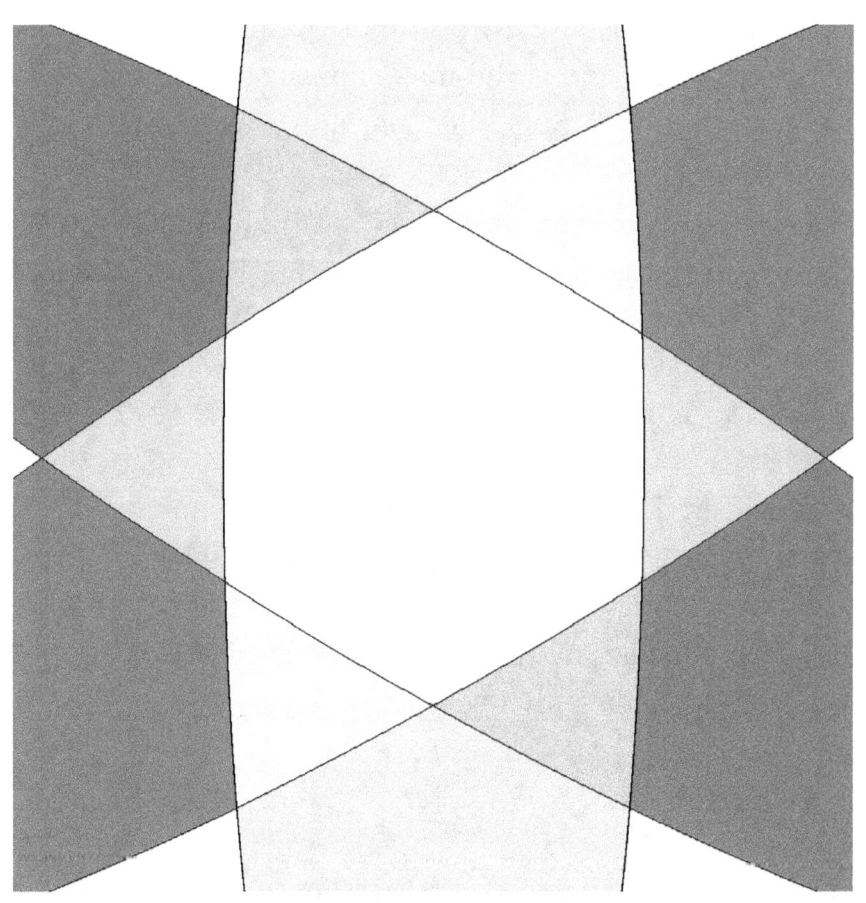

しかし、希望もあって、そんな酷（こく）な中でも、目には見えない感覚で感じる、世界も実在していて、やり方を間違えると、寒気や悪寒、さらには恐怖や不安を覚えるような苦しみを味わいます。

　However, there is hope, and even in such a harsh situation, there is a real world that you can feel in the invisible world, and if you make a mistake, you will experience the pain of chills, fear and anxiety.

　しかし、やり方さえ間違わなければ至福（しふく）と言いますか、極楽と言いますか、頭と心が共存する感覚とでも言いましょうか、心（ハート）と頭（マァーラ）が共存している感覚、体は脱力していて尚且（なおか）つ幸福感、至福感を味わい。天上の喜びを味わっているような様（さま）となりました。

　However, if you do it the right way, you can experience the feeling of bliss or paradise, where your heart and thoughts coexist. I am in a state of weakness. It is also a feeling of happiness and bliss. It was as if I was enjoying heavenly joy.

　その感覚を味わった時、これだ、これだ、これを味わっていたんだ。これを味わうためにアセンションを日々続けて来てたんだ。と弱気になっていた精神状態から回復して行く様（さま）を体感しています。

　When I tasted that feeling, I thought, this is it, this is it. In order to taste this, I have continued the rising air current (ascension) every day. I feel like I'm recovering from the mental state that was bearish.

しかし、ここで、重要になってくることがあります。理由はとかくわかりませんが、上昇気流（アセンション）を続けて行った結果、上昇気流（アセンション）依存症とも言えそうな状態へと移行していきます。

But here's where things become important. I don't know the reason, but as a result of continuing the ascending current, I will move to a state that can be said to be an ascending current (ascension) addiction.

　そうなってくると、自分の意思とは関係なく、上昇気流（アセンション）が立て続けに起こっていき、昼夜を問わず起こり狂うようになっていきます。こうなってくると、自分では手に負えないと判断してしまい病院を頼るようになっていきました。

When that happens, regardless of your will, the ascending current (ascension) will occur in quick succession, and it will be crazy regardless of the day or night. When this happened, I decided that I could not handle it by myself and started to rely on the hospital.

しかし、これには注意が必要です。お医者様は上昇気流（アセンション）体験をしたことない人達です。僕がいくら訴えても、頭のおかしいヤツにしか思いません。すぐに薬と療法に専念する話を持ちかけて来ます。僕は思いました。

But be careful with this. The doctors are people who have never had an ascension experience. No matter how much you complain to the doctor about the current situation, they will only think of you as a crazy person. I pondered.

自分に対して次のことを問いかけます。
Ask yourself:

あなたはアセンションを他人に理解出来るほどの説明力を持っていますか？僕の答えはNOでした。ですので、医者に頼っても答えは導き出されません。辛抱（しんぼう）強く自らの体と対話して対処法を構築して行くしか方法はございません。

Do you have the ability to explain the updraft (ascension) to others? My answer was NO. Therefore, even if you rely on the doctor, the answer will not be derived. There is no other way than to patiently interact with your own body and build a coping method.

しかし、現代であれば、その対処法は書物を通じて知り得ることができます。対策は可能ですし、少し良くなって、あの方法は正しいかどうかを検証していき、して良い方法と、してはならない方法の分別をつけて行くと、次第に答えが見えて来たりします。

However, in modern times, you can learn how to deal with it through books. Countermeasures are possible, and it gets a little better, and if you verify whether that method is correct or not, and if you make a distinction between what you should do and what you shouldn't do, you will gradually see the answer.

僕の場合、運良く本に恵まれ、運良く自分の生活パターン、思考パターン、行動パターンを検証することが出来ました。そういったことができるようになってくると、それまでの苦しみや寒気や悪寒や恐怖や不安などを少しづつ軽減できるようになり、冷静さを取り戻すに至（いた）りました。

In my case, fortunately, I was blessed with books, and fortunately, I was able to verify my life pattern, thought pattern, and behavior pattern. Once I was able to do that, I was able to gradually reduce the anguish, chills, fear, and anxiety I had until then, and regained my composure.

そして、わかってきたことがございます。どうやら、片方だけを上昇させると、閻魔［えんま］（王冠、豆）の判断によって、苦しみがもたらされ、寒気や悪寒、恐怖や不安が、表面化して苦しみを味わうようになっているようです。

And I have learned something. It seems that if only one side is raised, the judgment of Enma (crown, bean) will bring suffering, and chills, fears and anxieties will come to the surface and suffer.

片方だけではなく、両方を上昇させれば、なぜだかわからないですが、極上の至福、極楽を味わえるようになっているようです。

I don't know why, but if I raise both sides instead of just one, it seems that I can enjoy the ultimate bliss and paradise.

が、しかし、これからも検証は必要だと自認しながら評価すると、極楽と地獄は表裏一体となっていて、その者の持つ思考パターン、行動パターン、生活パターンによって、どちらにも転び得るようになっていると言うことだけ見えてきました。

However, when I evaluate it while admitting that I still need verification from now on, paradise and hell are two sides of the same coin, and depending on the person's thought pattern, behavior pattern, and life pattern, they can fall into either. I found out that.

僕が今、得ている、思考パターンを説明します。**目に見えないものを追いかけるようになったら、そのことにいち早く気づいて、目に見えるものを追いかける姿に戻ります。**と自らに宣言することです。

I'll explain the thought pattern I'm getting right now. If you start chasing something you can't see, you should be the first to notice it and declare to yourself, "I will return to chasing something visible."

これにより、過去の記憶に紐付（ひもづ）いた空想や妄想から脱却（だっきゃく）できます。また、反対のありもしない未来の空想や妄想からも脱却できます。

This allows you to escape from the fantasies and delusions associated with past memories. It also allows you to break away from the fantasies and delusions of the opposite non-existent future.

これは今は仮説ですが、いたずらに至福を望み、妙な空想や妄想をすることなく、ありのままの至福を味わい、腹八分目の極楽を享受できるようになるのではないかと考えているわけです。おそらく、その一線を越えると、苦しみや、寒気や悪寒、恐怖や不安を味わうようにできているのかもしれません。

This is just a hypothesis, but I believe that we will be able to enjoy the 80% paradise of the belly without wishing for bliss unnecessarily and without strange fantasies and delusions. Perhaps we are designed to experience suffering, chills and chills, fear and anxiety when we cross that line.

とりあえず、そう言うことが、少しわかってきたので、ご報告と説明をさせていただきます。

For the time being, I've come to understand a little about that, so I'll report and explain.

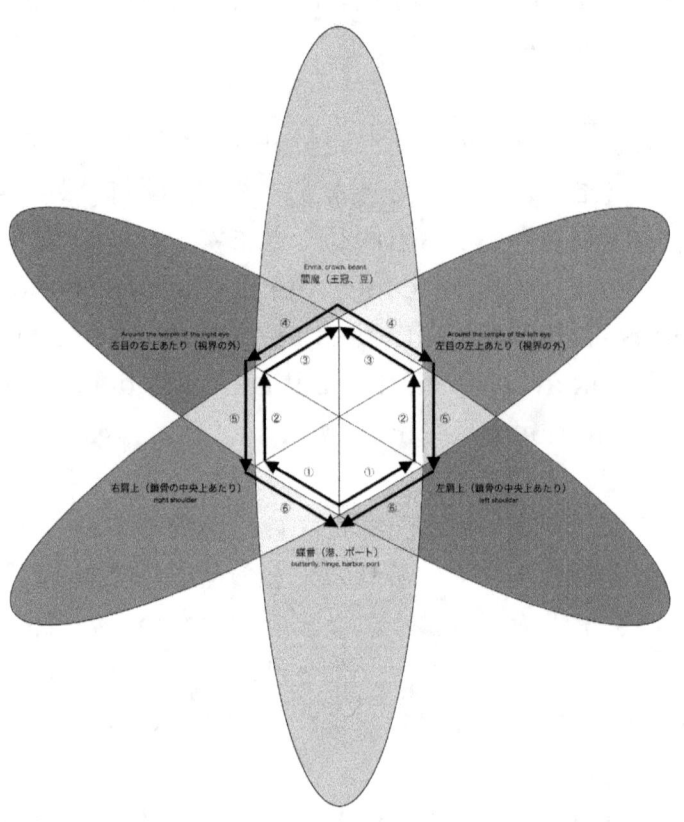

蝶番［ちょうつがい］部分（港やポートと書かれている部分）が出発点です。そして、左右の航路（こうろ）を同時にたどって行き、閻魔［えんま］部分（王冠、豆）と呼ばれる目的地に進んで行きます（数字表記で言う１、２、３を順に左右同時にたどっていきます）。

　The hinge part (the part written as harbor or port) is the starting point. Then, follow the left and right routes at the same time and proceed to the destination called the Enma part (crown, bean) (1, 2, 3 in numerical notation are followed at the same time on the left and right).

　これにより、ハートのエネルギーが頭のエネルギーへと意図的に上昇して行きます。そして、てっぺんまで行くと閻魔の判断を待ちます。閻魔の判断が出たら、左右の航路を同時にたどっていき、蝶番部分（港、ポート）へと戻って行きます（数字表記で言う４、５、６を順に左右同時にたどっていきます）。

　This intentionally moves the heart energy up into the head energy. And when you reach the top, you wait for Enma's judgment. When Enma makes a decision, follow the left and right routes at the same time and return to the hinge part (harbor, port). (4, 5, and 6 in numerical notation are traced in order at the same time on the left and right)

これにより、頭のエネルギーがハートのエネルギーへと意図的に下降して行きます。そして、極上の至福や極楽を味わうようになるのです。この方法を過（あやま）つと、苦しみ（寒気、悪寒、恐怖、不安）に変わるので注意が必要です。

This causes the energy of the head to intentionally descend into the energy of the heart. And you will come to taste the finest bliss and paradise. If you do not follow this method, it will turn into suffering (chills, fear, anxiety), so be careful.

　あっ、そうそう、蝶番（ちょうつがい）の部分（港、ポート）。その位置がどこにあるのか、これは、私の主観でお話をします。このままの書き方ではハートの中心のように取られてしまいかねません。心房（しんぼう）や心臓（しんぞう）と、とらえられがちかと思います。

Ah, yes, the hinge part (harbor, port). I will talk about where that position is based on my subjectivity. If you write it as it is, it may be taken like the center of the heart. I think we tend to think of it as the heart.

　が、しかし、私の感覚では、ちょっと上の方なんですね。

However, in my sense, it is a little higher position.

　感覚で感じる感覚が蝶（ちょう）みたいな感覚があるため蝶番（ちょうつがい）と表現して進めさせていただいています。

Since the feeling that I feel with my senses is like a butterfly, I express it as a hinge.

医学的な臓器（ぞうき）で説明すると、心臓の上あたりにある胸腺（きょうせん）なのではないかと私はとらえています。

In terms of organs expressed in the world of medicine, I believe it is the thymus located above the heart.

実際、目では確認できないところに、おもしろみがあります。

You can't see it with your eyes. The fun is hidden there.

また、閻魔［えんま］（王冠、豆）の部分。その位置がどこにあるのか、これも、私の主観でお話をします。王冠って表現すると、頭蓋骨（ずがいこつ）の頭頂骨（とうちょうこつ）と頭頂骨をつなぐ矢状縫合（しじょうほうごう）された広範囲な部分を連想されるかもしれないと思ったため、豆とも表現しています。

I thought that the crown might be associated with a wide circular part where the parietal bone and the parietal bone of the skull are sutured sagittal, so I dare to express it as a bean in order to express it with a dot.

豆は、上昇気流（アセンション）を続けていって、苦しみ抜いた先に現れ出でます。言葉では、まったく説明がつかないため、医学的な表現で説明すると、頭蓋骨（ずがいこつ）にある前頭骨（ぜんとうこつ）と左右の頭頂骨（とうちょうこつ）との間にある縫合（ほうごう）を冠状縫合（かんじょうほうごう）と呼びます。

Beans continue to rise (ascension) and appear at the end of their suffering. Words cannot explain it at all, so in medical terms, the suture between the frontal bone and the left and right parietal bones in the skull is called the coronal suture.

その冠状縫合（かんじょうほうごう）と矢状縫合（しじょうほうごう）が交わるポイントを豆の位置、閻魔［えんま］（王冠、豆）の位置と表現させて進めさせていただきます。

The point where the coronal suture and the sagittal suture intersect will be referred to as the position of the bean, or the position of Enma (crown, bean).

これも胸腺（きょうせん）と同様で、実際、目では確認できないところに、おもしろみがあります。

This is also similar to the thymus, and there is something interesting about it that cannot be seen with the naked eye.

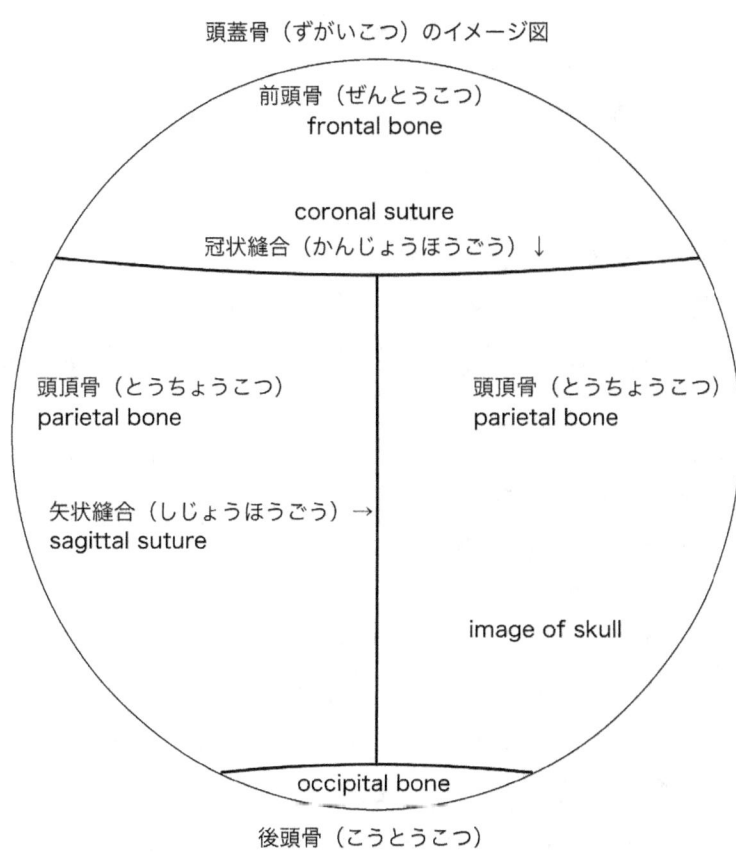

また、閻魔（えんま）と呼ぶ理由は、その王冠、豆の存在の判断を待（ま）つ行為（こうい）が、その昔読んだ西遊記やドラゴンボールなどに出てくる閻魔の絵図柄（えずがら）に酷似（こくじ）していたため、そう呼ばせていただいています。

　Also, the reason why it is called Enma is that the crown and the act of waiting for the bean's judgment is very similar to the image of Enma that appears in the Journey to the West and Dragon Ball, which I read long ago, so let me call it that.

　蝶番［ちょうつがい］（胸腺（きょうせん））から順をなして生命エネルギーが列を成して並んで昇（のぼ）っていく姿に、その物語たちが連想されて、よく似ていると思いました。

　The appearance of the life energy rising in a row from the hinge (thymus) in order reminds us of these stories, and is very similar. I thought.

　また、この呼び名は個人的主観であって、別の呼び名であってもいいと思っています。頭のてっぺんのことを最後の審判と呼ぼうが、胸の中心のことを港から出る箱舟と呼ぼうが、呼び名は、なんでもいいと思います。

　Also, this name is a personal subjectivity, and I think it can be another name. Whether you call the top of your head the Last Judgment, or the center of your chest the Ark out of the harbor, I think you can call it anything.

重要なのは、胸腺（蝶番、港、ポート）のエネルギーを左右両方から昇らせて、頭のてっぺん（閻魔、王冠、豆）の判断を待ち、判断が出てから、そのエネルギーを左右両方へと降ろしていき、故郷（ふるさと）でもある胸腺（蝶番、港、ポート）へとエネルギーを戻します。

　The important thing is to raise the energy of the thymus (hinge, harbor, port) from both left and right, wait for the judgment of the top of the head (Enma, crown, bean), and after the judgment is given, let the energy go down to both the left and right. and return the energy to the thymus (hinge, harbor, port), which is also the hometown.

　このことをポートランドやユートピアと呼んでも差し支（つか）えはないと自負（じふ）しております。また、呼び名について決め込まない方が後の人の世に栄光を与えるのではないかと考えています。
　I think it's safe to call this Portland or Utopia. Also, I think that it will give glory to the world of later generations if we do not prescribe names.

　こんなことを考えてるから、**目に見えないものを追い求めている姿となり、そのことに気が付いたならば、今こそ目に見えるものを追いかける姿に戻ります。**と、この文章を執筆しながら、宣言させていただきます。
　Because I'm thinking about this, I'm in the shape of pursuing something invisible. Once I realize that, I will declare as I write this sentence, "I will return to chasing the visible world."

このやり方であれば今のところ、問題なく極上の至福と言いますか、極楽を味わえています。とりあえず、安心している様子です。

With this method, so far, I can enjoy the finest bliss and paradise without any problems. For the time being, I feel safe.

　この記事を公開に踏み切った理由は、クリスタルヒーリングなどの上昇気流（アセンション）を助長させるヒーリングを学んで日々実践している人で、尚且（なおか）つ、上昇気流（アセンション）を体験していて、上昇気流（アセンション）依存症的な状況に苦悩している方がいたら、その方の解決策や救済策の一つとなれば、僕みたいに苦しまなくて済むのではないかと考えて公開に踏み切りました。

The reason I decided to publish this article is because I wanted to help people who are suffering from symptoms of ascension addiction.

　また、上昇気流（アセンション）と表現せずに、ヨーガの世界ではクンダリーニの上昇と呼ばれていたりもします。ですから、クンダリーニ症候群などでお困りの方の解決策や、救済策となれれば本望です。

Also, instead of expressing it as an ascending current, it is sometimes called the ascension of the Kundalini in the world of yoga. Therefore, it is my sincere hope that it can be a solution or a remedy for those who are in trouble with Kundalini syndrome.

また、これを機に上昇気流（アセンション）に興味が湧（わ）かれた方がいらっしゃいましたら、まず一つ、忠告（ちゅうこく）をさせていただきます。通常、上昇気流（アセンション）を説明されている方は快楽が得られるんだと、主張して勧誘（かんゆう）をしています。または、至福を味わってみないかと誘（さそ）いがかかるかもしれません。

　Also, if you are interested in the updraft (ascension) on this occasion, I would like to give you one piece of advice. When preaching healing like this, there are cases where you are soliciting by claiming that you can get pleasure. Or you may be tempted by being touted as a way to get bliss.

　が、しかし、注意が必要です。その快楽と引き換えに極上の地獄も用意されています。生死を彷徨（さまよ）う絵図らもようともなりかねないため、正直、上昇気流（アセンション）させる方法を気安く人におすすめする気はございません。

　But be careful. In exchange for that pleasure, the finest hell is also prepared. To be honest, I don't feel comfortable recommending the method of ascension to people because it can be a picture of life and death.

　経験上、おすすめする気にもなれません。
　Based on my experience, I wouldn't recommend it.

ですから、上昇気流（アセンション）を助長するような、作法を行っていった先には、寒気や悪寒や恐怖感や不安感などを味わってしまい生死を賭（か）けた展望へと誘（いざ）われてしまいます。その地獄を味わってでも極上の至福を味わってみたいと思われる方であれば良いのですが、そうでないのであれば、絶対に手を出さない方が得策です。

If you follow a method that promotes the updraft (ascension), you will experience chills, fear, and anxiety, and will be invited to a life-and-death prospect. If you want to experience hell and get bliss, it's fine, but if you don't, it's better to never get involved.

　ここは念をおして言っておきます。
　Please take it as advice.

また、それでも上昇気流（アセンション）体験をしてみたい方がいらっしゃいましたら、地獄を味わう覚悟と、一切の責任はお客様自身にあることをここに明記して進ませていただきます。

Also, if you still want to experience the ascending air current (ascension), we will clearly state that you are prepared to experience hell and that all responsibility lies with you.

また、その後に起こるお客様の身体への保証は一切致しません。お客様の自己判断で自己責任でお進みくださればと思います。

In addition, we do not guarantee any damage to the customer's body after that. We ask that you proceed at your own discretion and at your own risk.

上昇気流（アセンション）させる方法を今回ご紹介しますが、私 Mr. Takashi 2baki は、ご紹介する作法によって生まれる、ありとあらゆる現象に対しての一切の責任を負いません。予めご了承ください。お客様の自己責任でお願いします。

I, Mr. Takashi 2baki, will not be held responsible for any and all phenomena caused by the methods I introduce. Please note. Please do so at your own risk.

このことを同意頂けた方のみ、先へお進みください。
Please proceed only if you agree to this.

まえがき
FOREWORD

※注意事項：上昇気流（アセンション）が頭蓋（ずがい）の中まで起こるようになって来ますと、精神的に朦朧（もうろう）とした状態となります。起きてるのか眠ってるのか、よく判（わか）らない状態となり、瞑想（めいそう）しなくても瞑想している様な状態を体験します。

*Caution: When the rising air current (ascension) begins to occur in the skull, it will be in a state of mental drowsiness (sleeping). You will not know if you are awake or asleep, and you will experience a state of meditation even if you do not meditate.

また、上昇気流（アセンション）のやり方を間違えてしまっている場合や、やってはいけない作法をしている状態（思考パターン、行動パターン、生活パターンなど）の場合や、特に初めての体験の場合は、寒気や悪寒や恐怖感や不安感を自ら作り出しやすい状態となっていきます。

Also, if you have made a mistake in how to ascend, or if you are doing something that should not be done (thinking pattern, action pattern, life pattern, etc.), especially if it is your first experience, you may experience chills or You will be in a state of self-creating chills, fear, and anxiety.

多感で敏感（びんかん）で些細（ささい）なことにでも反応してしまう体の状態となり、心も体もバランスを崩（くず）しやすい状態になっていく可能性がございます。この状態になりますと特に注意が必要です。

It is possible that your body will become sensitive and sensitive, reacting to even trivial things, and that your mind and body will become easily out of balance. Special care must be taken in this situation.

本編 MAIN STORY

　これより、上昇気流（アセンション）をスムーズに進めるためのヒーリングの仕方をご紹介します。焦（あせ）らずにゆっくりと進めて行くことを推奨（すいしょう）しております。実際に、お客様が閻魔（えんま）の話にたどり着くまでには幾多（いくた）の年月がかかることになります。僕の話をするとヒーリングを始めて、ちょうど２年と１０ヶ月かかっております。ですので、３年はかかると思っていただいて結構です。

　From here, we will introduce how to heal to smoothly advance the ascending air current (ascension). We recommend that you proceed slowly without rushing. In fact, it will take many years for customers to reach the story of Enma. From my experience, it took 2 years and 10 months. Therefore, it is fine to think that it will take three years.

　また、最初の上昇気流（アセンション）が起こるようになるまでにも、幾月（いくつき）か時間がかかります。
　It will also take several months for the first updrafts (ascension) to occur.

　僕の場合で、３ヶ月から半年かかっております。ですので、気長に続けて行かれることをおすすめします。
　For me, it took 3 to 6 months. Therefore, I recommend that you keep going.

また、この時に必要となる力（ちから）が三つほどございます。それは、見えたり聞こえたり感じたりする感覚を抗（あらが）わずに進んで体験していく想像力と。今、この体に何が起きているのかを注意して感じ取り観察して見ていく観察力と。継続（けいぞく）してヒーリングを続けていける並々ならぬ熱意とも呼ばれる熱中力です。この三つがあれば、きっと、たどり着けることでしょう。

　Also, there are three powers that are needed at this time. It is the imagination that willingly experiences the sensations of seeing, hearing, and feeling without resisting. The power of observation to observe what is happening in this body. Enthusiasm that can be called extraordinary enthusiasm to continue healing while enjoying it. With these three things, you'll definitely get there.

　上昇気流（アセンション）が起こるようになってからは、その現象に、ときめくことになると思います。すっごく初々（ういうい）しく楽しい時期に入って行きますので、いっぱい楽しんであげてください。

　After the rising air current (ascension) begins to occur, I think that the phenomenon will make your heart flutter. It's going to be a really fresh and fun time, so please enjoy it to the fullest.

それでは、基本となるヒーリングを伝授します。
Now, let me teach you the basics of healing.

今回は特別に私が伝授を受けたそのままの原文でご紹介、差し上げます。
This time, I will introduce and give you the original text that I received the instruction.

クリスタルヒーリング
CRYSTAL HEALING

クリスタルヒーリングの伝承者はこう語られました。
A person who taught me crystal healing told me this.

あなたの惹（ひ）かれるクリスタル（石）を選んで下さい。そして深い呼吸をして、目を閉じて、その石を私のハートに持っていきます。あなたのハートに両手であてがって下さい。
Please choose the crystal (stone) that you are attracted to. Then I take a deep breath, close my eyes and bring the stone to my heart. Place both hands on your heart.

息を吸うときには、石の存在に、どうぞお越（こ）し下さい。と言ってハートに歓迎（かんげい）する気持ちで迎（むか）え入れます。息を吐くときには私がこの石の存在の方に、抱（いだ）く愛と友情を、どうぞ、お受け取り下さい。と言って与えます。

As you breathe in, please come to the inner being that resides within the stone. I will welcome you with a feeling of welcoming with my heart. As I exhale, I give the love and friendship that I have to the inner being that resides within this stone by saying, "Please take it."

そして、数回呼吸をするごとに、今の気持ちの交流をやります。何度も繰り返すうちにエネルギーが循環しているというのがだんだん感じてきますので、それまで、呼吸をして、気持ちを伝えていきます。

Then, with each breath, exchange your current feelings. As you repeat it over and over, you will gradually feel that the energy is circulating, so continue to convey your feelings while breathing.

で、その石の存在の方を歓迎（かんげい）するのと同じくらい重要で、石に対して、愛の気持ちと、感謝の気持ちを捧（ささ）げるというのは、とても重要なことです。

It is very important to offer love and gratitude to the stone. It is as important as welcoming the presence of the stone.

なぜ、重要かと言いますと、この愛と感謝の気持ちというのは、それによって石が滋養（じよう）を受けるのですね。栄養を受け取ります。愛と感謝の気持ちというのは、地球に対しても大変良いメリットを与えます。栄養を与えることになるのです。

The reason why it is important is that this feeling of love and gratitude nourishes the stone. The stone receives nourishment. Feelings of love and gratitude are also very beneficial to the planet. It will nourish the earth.

その気持ちを持って交流していくと、だんだん、そのエネルギーが大きくなっていきます。そうすると、向こうからもフィードバックして、その都度（つど）に加算されて、その都度（つど）に大きくなっていきます。

If you interact with the stone with that feeling, the energy will gradually increase. Then, feedback from the other side is added each time, and it grows bigger each time.

そして、サーキュレーションして大きくなってくると、渦巻状（うずまきじょう）に大きくなってきて、アセンションするためのパターンの一つが出来上がります。まもなく、この石の存在の方と共に瞑想（めいそう）します。そして、その存在と出会って感じていただくというのをやります。

And as it circulates and grows, it spirals out and forms one of the patterns for Ascension. Soon you will meditate with this stone being. And I will do it to meet and feel that existence.

そして、先程のように呼吸しながら、気持ちを伝えて、その都度（つど）エネルギーを受け取り、与えて、それをハートでやっているうちに、だんだん、石の存在がハートの中にきて、ハートの中でイメージを見せてくれることがありますので、それを体験してみて下さい。

Then, while breathing like before, convey your feelings, receive and give energy each time, and do it with your heart, gradually the presence of the stone will come into your heart. There are things that show you the image in your heart, so please experience it.

で、その石の存在のイメージがハートの中で見えてきたら、質問をします。「あなたの本質、性質はどういうものですか？そして、私はあなたと一緒にどういうことを共に生み出していくことが出来ますか？」

Then, when you see the image of the existence of the stone in your heart, ask a question. "What is your nature and what can I co-create with you?"

で、その時の石の存在からの返答というのは、何かを見せてくれるかもしれません。何かを見せられるかもしれません。本人の姿という形でイメージを送ってくるかもしれません。あるいわ、お願いします。と言ったら、だんだん、こう景色が変わってジャーニーの旅路に、いろんなところに連れていってくれるかもしれません。

So, the response from the existence of the stone at that time may show us something. I may be able to show you something in the form of a reply from a stone being. They may send you images in the form of who they are. Or if you say "Please", the scenery will gradually change and you may be taken to various places on your journey.

そして、イメージ、もしくは、ヒーリング、感覚でこんな感じってのが来た時というのは、自分でこさえないで、だんだん大きくなるように、もっと見せてください。という感じで、委（ゆだ）ねて、大きく強くさせていってください。そして、起きたことはメモにとると良いでしょう。

And when an image, or a feeling of healing, comes to me, I don't resist, but gradually entrust it with the feeling of "Please show me more" and make it bigger and stronger. please And make a note of what happened.

それでは、目を閉じて、用意をします。そして、呼吸に集中、石をハートのあたりに置いて下さい。ハーっと息を吐きワークを開始して下さい。

Now close your eyes and get ready. Then focus on your breath and place the stone around your heart. Take a deep breath and start working.

瞑想（めいそう）を終わらせる時は、石の存在達に感謝を伝えましょう。感謝が終わったら、ゆっくりと整えてこちらにお戻り下さい。
End your meditation by thanking the stone beings. When you have finished thanking you, please slowly prepare and return here.

終わったら、忘れないうちにメモをとると良いでしょう。私の本はこのメモから作られています。
When you're done, it's a good idea to take notes before you forget. My book is made from this memo.

今の体験によってハートに良い感覚が来た方はいらっしゃいますか？
Is there anyone who has had a good feeling in their heart from this experience?

このハートの中で感じている、良い感覚は、深い自己、ディープセルフが動き出している、その感覚なんです。
The good feeling that you are feeling in this heart is that feeling that your deep self, your deep self, is in motion.

そして、特に重要となるのが、次のヒーリングです。
And the next healing is especially important.

深い自己、ディープセルフと出会うというプロセスを行っていただきます。
You will go through the process of encountering your deep self.

深い自己（ディープセルフ）との出会い方
HOW TO MEET YOUR DEEP SELF

クリスタルヒーリングの伝承者はこう語られました。
A person who taught me crystal healing told me this.

ハートの中に洞穴（ほらあな）が口を開けているイメージを見てください。洞穴の口から下に下降していくようになります。どんどん下に降りて行って底辺のところまで降りて行ってください。

See the image of the cave opening into the heart. It will start descending from the mouth of the cave. Keep going down and down until you reach the bottom.

そして、底辺までたどり着いたら、周りを見渡してください。わずかな光がそこにあります。じーっと見ていると扉が見えてきます。扉を見ているとあなたの名前が書いてあります。その扉が見つかったらノックしてください。扉を開いて中に入ります。

And when you get to the bottom, look around. I can see a faint light. If you look closely, you can see the door. You will see a door with your name on it. Knock on the door when you find it. Open the door and go inside.

そこに誰かが立っています。あなたの内側の深い自己。この存在と出会いましたら、あなたの愛と友情を提供して差し上げてください。そして、あなたのハートの底辺にある扉を開けてくれてありがとうと伝えてください。

someone is standing there. your inner deep self. Offer your love and friendship when you meet this being. And say thank you for opening the door at the bottom of your heart.

そして、その方に質問をします。私に何をお伝えしたいですか？そして、そのことに関して、私には、何ができますか？と聞いてください。
And question its existence. Ask, "What do you want me to tell you?" And for that matter, "What can I do?"

その後に何が起ころうと、抗（あらが）うことなく委（ゆだ）ねて起こるがままにしてください。
Whatever happens after that, let it happen without resistance.

そして、あなたは来た道をたどって、ハートのところまで戻っていき、休憩をしてください。
And follow the way you came. Let's go back to the "heart". And take a break.

それでは、石をハートのところまで持ってきてクリスタルヒーリングをする準備をしてください。あなたはハートから洞穴（ほらあな）、下向きな洞穴を下がってあなたのハートの奥底にいる深い自己、ディープセルフと出会います。
Now bring the stone to your heart and get ready for crystal healing. You go down from the heart into the cave, the downward cave, to meet the Deep Self in the depths of your heart.

それでは、クリスタルヒーリングを開始してください。
Now let the crystal healing begin.

終わりましたら、整えてからこちらへお戻りください。
When you're done, clean up your mind and come back here.

洞穴から降りて行って深い自己、ディープセルフと出会えましたか？これこそ私が出来うる中で最も重要なヒーリングだと思います。このことをすることによって、深い自己、ディープセルフが浮上して来て、あなたと一緒に生きていくということができるようになるでしょう。
Did you go down from the cave and meet your deep self? I believe this is the most important healing I can do. By doing this, you will allow your deep self to come to the surface and live with you.

自分と深い自己、ディープセルフが実は一つの存在なんだという風に感じることが出来るかもしれません。このかけのない全体像が取れたとき、日常生活の中で深い自己、ディープセルフと共に生きていくことができるようになります。
You may feel that you and your deep self are actually one entity. When you get this complete picture, you will be able to live with your deep self in your daily life.

深い自己、ディープセルフと合体して一つになることが必要なんです。大抵の場合、深い自己、ディープセルフとつながったら、自分の手にするということが起こります。

You need to merge and become one with your Deep Self. Most of the time, what happens is that when you connect with your Deep Self, you get your hands on it.

ですけれども、見失うことがあります。そして、戻って来てくれる。そういうことが起こります。
But sometimes you lose sight of it. and will come back. That kind of thing happens.

もし深い自己、ディープセルフを見失った場合は、また、洞穴（ほらあな）の中に入って行って、また出会うということをしていただければ、また出会うことができます。
If you lose sight of your deep self, you can find it again by going into the cave and meeting again.

それでは、次に、普段、僕が行っているヒーリングをご紹介します。これは、先にご紹介したクリスタルヒーリングのクリスタルを外したバージョンのヒーリングとなります。わたくしごとではありますが、ここ２年くらいはこっちのヒーリングをメインに上昇気流（アセンション）を行ってきました。

Next, I will introduce the healing that I usually do. This is a version of healing without the crystals. For the past two years, I have been doing this healing and causing an updraft (ascension).

愛と友情のエネルギーの使い方
USING LOVE AND FRIENDSHIP ENERGY

若き日のあなたにお伝え申します。ハートの中心に両手が重なり合うようにあてがってください。どちらの手が上か下かは、あなたが心地よいと思う方を選んでください。

Place both hands on top of each other in the center of the heart.

それでは、息をふぅ〜っと吐き出してください。息を吐き出しきったら、素早く息を吸い込み、ゆっくり息を吐き出しながら、自己に内在する存在に伝えていきます。

Then, please exhale. When you have finished exhaling, inhale quickly and exhale slowly as you communicate to the existence within yourself.

自己に内在する存在である、
あなた様に愛と友情をささげます。
わたしはあなた様を愛しております。
わたしはあなた様と友達です。
I offer my love and friendship to you,
the being that is inherent in me.
I love you
I am friends with you.

　これを息継ぎのたびに繰り返していきます。今のあなたに時間的余裕があるなら、そのまま瞑想をしましょう。
　Repeat this with each breath. If you have time now, let's meditate as it is.

　※特に瞑想する時間に決まりはありません。あなたの赴（おもむ）くままに心地よいだけ行っていただけたらと思います。
　*Meditation time is free. I would like you to go as comfortable as you want.

　ハートの中心より出でてまいります、愛と友情のエネルギーの感覚を感じられた方はいらっしゃいますか？または、イメージやビジョン、サウンドやミュージック、動画や物語など、様々な形で何かを見せてくれるかもしれません。
　Can any of you feel the energy of love and friendship emanating from the center of your heart? Or they may show us something in various forms, such as images, sounds, stories, etc.

そんな感覚、感じがきたら、自分でこさえないで、もっと見せてくださいと言うように、あらがわずに進んで体験していきましょう。これは自己に内在する存在が動き出しているその証拠なんです。

If you feel that way, don't hold back and go ahead and experience it as if you want to see more. This is the proof that the existence inherent in the self is starting to move.

また、愛と友情のエネルギーの使い方をして起きたことは忘れないうちにメモにとっておきましょう。

Also, make a note of what happens when you use the energy of love and friendship before you forget it.

僕の本はこのメモから作られています。

My book is made from this memo.

以上で、ヒーリングのご紹介を終わります。僕は、先にご紹介した、クリスタルヒーリングを約半年間続けたことにより上昇気流（アセンション）体験をしました。アセンションを日本語で言うと上昇気流が体に感じられるレベルで起こったと言えます。
　This concludes the introduction to healing. As I introduced earlier, I had an ascension experience by continuing the crystal healing for about half a year. In Japanese, we can say that the updraft occurred at a level that can be felt in the body.

　そして、それを飽きずに２年と１０ヶ月続けた結果、本書の最初にご紹介した現象にまで、たどり着くことが出来ました。クリスタルヒーリングを伝授してくれた伝承者様のことを心から感謝しております。
　And as a result of continuing it for 2 years and 10 months without getting tired of it, I was able to reach the phenomenon introduced at the beginning of this book. I would like to express my sincere gratitude to those who taught me crystal healing.

　また、このヒーリングを半年間継続しても上昇気流（アセンション）が起こらなかった場合の対策として一つの呼吸法をご紹介して本編を締（し）めくくらせていただきます。
　In addition, I would like to conclude the main part by introducing one breathing method as a countermeasure in the case that an ascending current (ascension) does not occur even after continuing this healing for half a year.

この呼吸法は、まだ上昇気流（アセンション）の文字も知らない頃、今から１０年くらい前に、たまたま読んだ本の中にあった呼吸法を実践していた時に起こった不思議体験です。

　This breathing method is a strange experience that happened to me about 10 years ago when I was practicing a breathing method that I happened to read in a book when I didn't even know the word for ascending current (ascension).

　これが、もしや、その後の、上昇気流（アセンション）に関係しているかもしれないと思っての情報提供となります。必ずしも、この呼吸法をしなければ上昇気流（アセンション）できないと言うわけではありません。あくまで、上記に記述したヒーリングを半年間試してみても、なにも起きなかった人用にご提供、差し上げたいと思います。

　This is the information that I think that it may be related to the rising air current (ascension) after that. It doesn't necessarily mean that you can't "ascend" without this breathing technique. I would like to offer and give it to those who have tried the healing described above for half a year and nothing happened.

昔、やった呼吸法
BREATHING METHOD

　確か、あれは、３０代前半の頃、今 {2022/05/31} から８年〜１０年くらい前のこと、正確には覚えていません。
　Certainly, it was around 8 to 10 years ago from now when I was in my early 30s, so I don't remember exactly.

　ヨガや自己啓発本のたぐいを読み漁（あさ）っていました、呼吸で体調が変わるみたいな本がいくつかあって、その中のどれかに、息を限りなく長く吐くことに集中した呼吸法があり、ただひたすら、息を長く吐く練習をしていました。
　I was reading all sorts of yoga and self-help books, and there were several books that seemed to change your physical condition with your breath, and one of them had a breathing technique that focused on long exhalations. It was just a practice of exhaling long breaths earnestly.

　確か、やり方は、口を半開きにして、舌を上顎（うわあご）につけて、息を少しづつ吐く様にして、吐く時間を少しづつ長くしていく方法でした。
　If I remember correctly, the method was to open the mouth halfway, put the tongue on the upper jaw, exhale little by little, and gradually lengthen the exhalation time.

初めの頃は４秒吐きを繰り返し、出来る様になってきたら８秒に切り替えて、少しづつ時間を長くしていき、１０秒、１５秒、３０秒、と続けていき、確か、６０秒くらいまで長く吐ける様になって、それをどれくらい繰り返せるか、みたいな挑戦的なことをやっていた時のこと、急に、吐く息と吸う息が同時に起こり、なんじゃこりゃぁって驚（おどろ）きながら面白がって笑っていたことがあったなぁと思い出しました。

In the beginning, repeat exhaling for 4 seconds, then switch to 8 seconds when you can do it, and gradually increase the time, 10 seconds, 15 seconds, 30 seconds, and so on, and if I remember correctly, about 60 seconds. I was able to exhale for a long time, and when I was doing something challenging like how many times I could repeat it, suddenly, exhaling and inhaling occurred at the same time, and I was surprised and amused. I remembered that I was laughing.

　今、やれって言われても出来る気はしませんが、その当時、驚（おどろ）いたのを覚えています。確か、その時、臍下（へそした）あたりが気持ちよくなっていたなぁと思い返します。

I don't think I can do it now, but I remember being surprised at the time. I remember that at that time, I felt comfortable around the navel.

　今から思うと、あれって、もしかしたら、その後に起こる上昇気流（アセンション）体験に一役かってたんじゃないのかなぁ、と、今更（いまさら）ながらに思い始めています。

Thinking back on it now, I'm starting to think that maybe it played a part in the experience of the updraft (ascension) that would follow.

特に科学的な根拠はありませんが、もしかしたら、っと思っての情報提供となります。
There is no particular scientific basis, but it is possible to provide information.

それでは、これをもって、本編を締（し）めくくらせていただきたいと思います。拝読（はいどく）頂き誠にありがとうございました。あなた様に光のある日が訪れることを心からお祈りしております。ではでは。
With that, I would like to conclude this volume. Thank you very much for reading. I pray from the bottom of my heart that a bright day will come to you. See you soon.

引用・参考文献一覧
LITERATURE LIST

素直な心になるために（著者）松下幸之助
To become an obedient heart (Author) Konosuke Matsushita

人間を考える（著者）松下幸之助
Thinking about Humans (Author) Konosuke Matsushita

復職後再発率ゼロの心療内科の先生に「薬に頼らず、うつを治す方法」を聞いてみました 亀廣 聡（著）夏川 立也（著）
I asked a psychosomatic doctor who has zero recurrence rate after returning to work, "How to cure depression without relying on drugs" Satoshi Kamehiro (Author) Tatsuya Natsukawa (Author)

武術格闘家 菊野克紀 の 誰ツヨDOJOy
Martial arts fighter Katsunori Kikuno's who Tsuyo DOJOy
https://www.youtube.com/watch?v=8H6LtlSZ8Bw

良い音は、良い姿勢、良い呼吸でつくられる（著者）眞々田昭司

Good sound is made with good posture and good breathing (Author) Shoji Mamada

Special Thanks : ロバート・シモンズ Robert Simmons

作者について
ABOUT THE AUTHOR

　西暦1981年に日本に生まれ、つばきたかしと命名される。高校を卒業と同時に上京して電気技術者になる。途中でプログラミングに目覚めプログラマーに転身しIT企業に転職をする。インターネットが完全に普及したタイミングで故郷に移住して地元の企業に転職する。転職に転職を重ねていく間に好きなことを仕事にするというビジョンに触れ勢い良く整っていくネットビジネスの環境を鑑みて一念発起して自作自演のミュージシャンになる。しかし、思ったような成果が出ず、流れが変わって、大好きな天然石をビジネスにしようと考えて、プランBとして天然石shopを始める。そうこうしているうちに、運が巡り廻ってきてクリスタルヒーリングの伝承者に直接会う機会を得て、直々にクリスタルヒーリングを伝授される。それ以来、執筆活動をしています。

　Born in Japan in 1981 AD and named Takashi 2baki. Upon graduating from high school, he moved to Tokyo to become an electrical engineer. He awakens to programming on the way, turns into a programmer and changes jobs to an IT company. At the timing when the Internet became completely popular, he moved to his hometown and changed jobs to a local company. While changing jobs repeatedly, he came into contact with the vision of doing what he likes as a job, and in view of the Internet business environment, which was rapidly developing, he made up his mind to become a self-produced musician. However, he didn't get the results he expected, and the trend changed, so he decided to turn his favorite natural stone into a business, and started a natural stone shop as Plan B. In the meantime, he got lucky and got an opportunity to meet the person who taught him crystal healing, and he was taught crystal healing directly. Since then, I have been working on writing.

Mr. Takashi 2baki

https://note.com/mr_takashi_2baki/

おまけ BONUS

　ひとえに両方を上昇させるといっても様々な上昇のさせ方が現れてきます。僕の場合、心の虫の音と言いますか、スピリットガイドと言いますか、うちなる声、自己に内在する存在の声、うちなるガイダンスに従った形で上昇の仕方が日々変わってきています。そのことを踏まえた上で、その中でも良かったなぁ。と思える上昇パターンをご紹介します。

　Even if you simply raise both, there are various ways to raise it. In my case, the way I ascend is changing day by day in accordance with the inner voice, the voice of the being that resides within me, the inner guidance, the sound of the bugs in my heart, or the spirit guide. With that in mind, it was good. I'd like to introduce you to the rising pattern that seems to be.

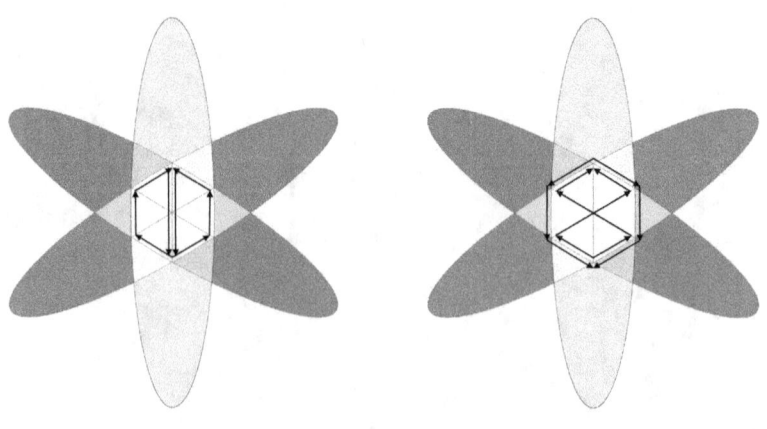

また、良きことがあった日の上昇の仕方も記述します。
It also describes how the ascension was when good things happened.

　参考資料となれば幸いです。
I hope that it will be useful as a reference material.

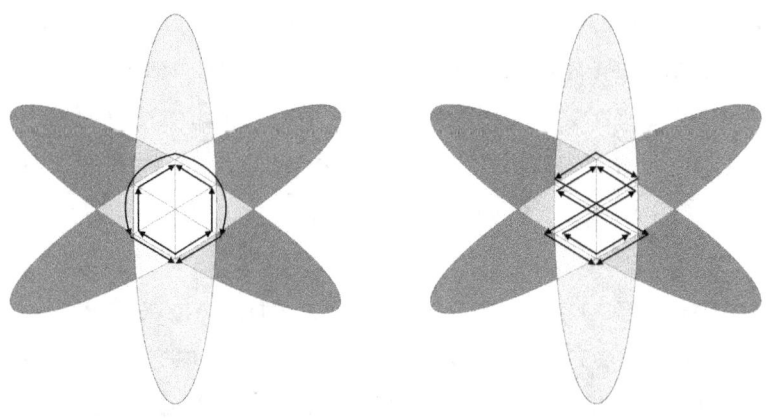

つばきたかし画伯の絵（１）［エネルギーの道］
Painting by 2baki Takashi (1) [Energy Road]

　覚醒体験へと移り進んでいく最中（さなか）、２０２２年５月中旬頃に起きたことを簡略的にイメージ図にしてまとめてみました。細かい詳細は秘密とさせていただきます。秘密にする理由は、名前などの名称や細かい順序などの詳細は、人によって呼び名やエネルギーの道そのものが変わってくる可能性があるからです。おそらく昇り方も変わってくるでしょうし、見え方や感じ方、とらえ方も人によって変わってくると思います。また名前などを明示したり開示したりすると、お客様がその名前の影響を受けてしまって、お客様自身の体得の邪魔をしてしまいかねません。その影響を最小限にするためにも、名前や名称や呼び名などの細かい詳細は秘密とさせていただきます。覚醒体験へと導かれていく最中に、こんなことがあったよ程度に見ていただけたら幸いです。

　I have put together a simplified image of what happened around mid-May 2022 during the transition to the awakening experience. The finer details will be kept confidential. The reason for keeping it secret is that details such as names and detailed orders may change the names and energy paths themselves depending on the person. The way it climbs will probably change, and the way it looks and perceives it will also change depending on the person. Also, if you specify or disclose your name, etc., the customer will be influenced by that name, and it may interfere with your own experience. In order to minimize the impact, detailed details such as names, designations, and nicknames will be kept confidential. It seems that something like this happened while being led to the awakening experience. I would appreciate it if you could see it to that extent.

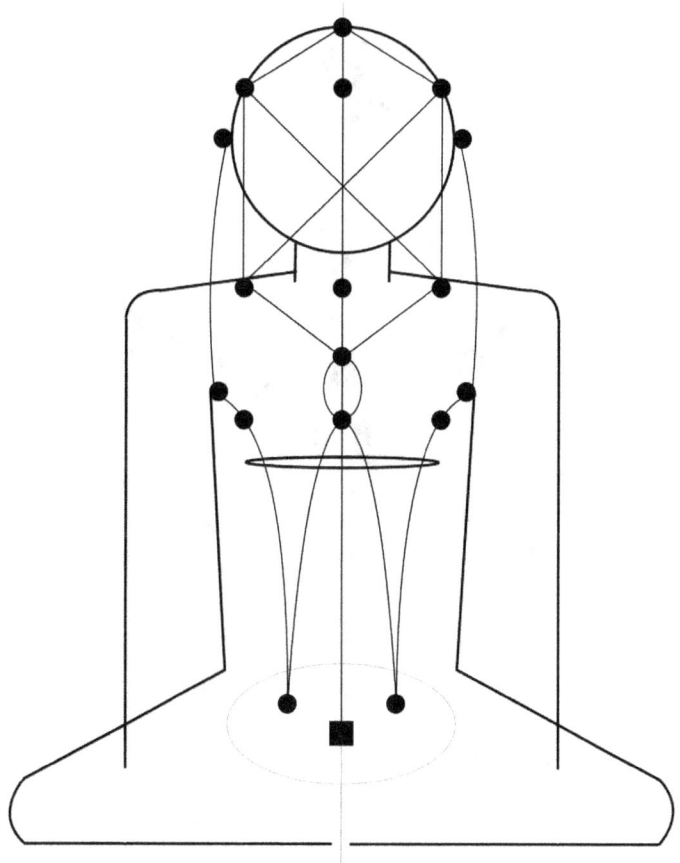

つばきたかし画伯の絵（2）［月と太陽と己の光］
Painting by Takashi 2baki (2) [The Moon, the Sun and My Light]

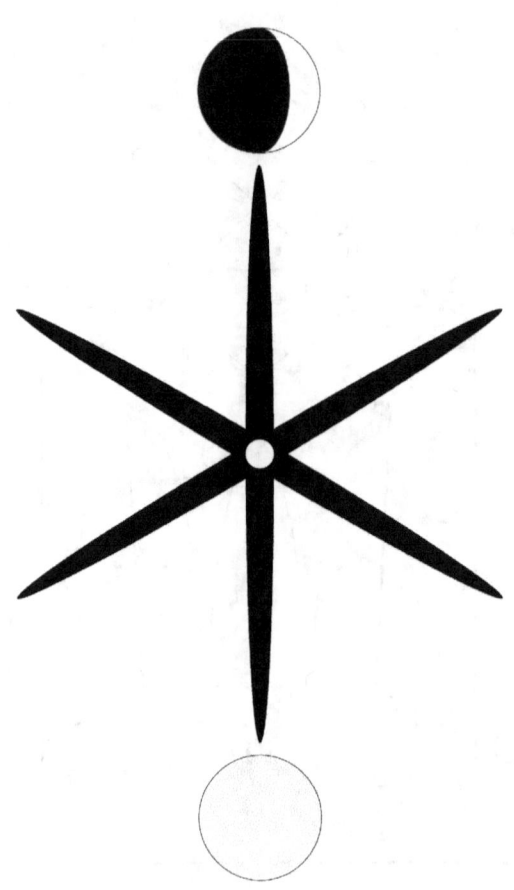

地獄の苦しみの最中、覚醒体験へ突入して行く流れの中で、六芒星（ろくぼうせい）の明示があった後、明示された言葉があって、その言葉を元に描いたイメージ図です。深い意味は考えずに絵画をお楽しみいただければ幸いです。

　In the midst of hellish suffering, in the flow of rushing into the awakening experience, after the hexagram was clarified, there was a clarified word, and it is an image drawing based on that word. I hope you can enjoy the paintings without thinking about the deep meaning.

ペンデュラムの使い方
How to use the pendulum

　伝承者はこう答えられました。ペンデュラムの使い方、動きは、いつも自分のディープセルフに聞いてみるんですね。「YES（イエス）のときの動きを私に見せてください」というように聞いてみて、どちらの方向にどの様に動くのか観察してみます。そして、「どっちの方向にどのように動くのがNO（ノー）なのですか」とディープセルフに聞いてみます。すると、YES（イエス）の時とNO（ノー）の時の違いが現れてくると思います。そして、その動き方は人それぞれ違います。

　This is what the person who taught me crystal healing said. I always ask my deep self how to use the pendulum and how to move it. Try asking something like, "Show me how it moves when you say YES," and observe how it moves in which direction. Then, ask the deep self, "Which direction and how is it 'NO' to move?" Then, I think that the difference between YES and NO will appear. And how it moves varies from person to person.

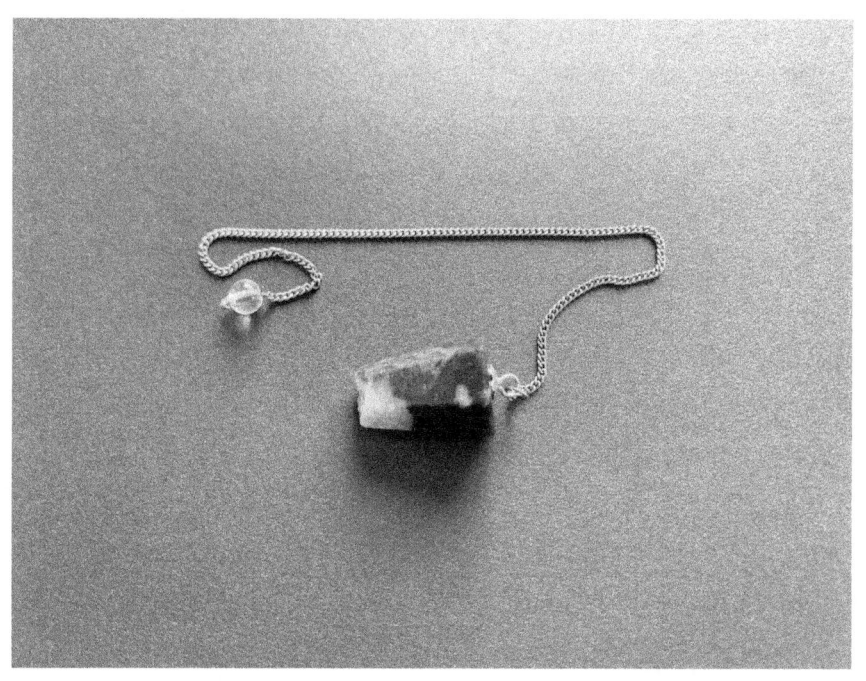

光の三原色、色の三原色、ひかりのしるし。
The three primary colors of light, the three primary colors of color, and the sign of light.

　量子理論の中にある目に見える光（可視光線）を勉強していたところ、白と黒が無いなぁという疑問から、光の三原色にたどりつき、緑と、青と、赤が、混ざると白になる。と言うことを知りました。

　When I was studying visible light in quantum theory, I came to the three primary colors of light from the question that white and black do not exist. If you mix green, blue and red, you get white.

　また、黒は、色の三原色と呼ばれ、光の三原色で出て来た各々の色同士が混じり合った三色（緑と青が混ざったシアン［水色に近い青緑色］、青と赤が混ざったマゼンタ［明るく鮮やかな赤紫色］、赤と緑が混ざったイエロー［黄色］）が混ざり合うと黒になると言うことを知りました。

　Also, black is called the three primary colors of color, and is a mixture of the three primary colors of light. Cyan is a mixture of green and blue, magenta is a mixture of blue and red, and yellow is a mixture of red and green. I learned that when these three colors are mixed, they become black.

考えれば考えるほど、なぜだって思いが強くなる白と黒です。が、しかし、色は波だと考えて、黒は波が打ち消しあって発光しないから黒に見えるのかな、白は反対に波が乱れ合って発光するから白に見えるのかな、そういった解釈をしています。

The more I think about it, the more I wonder why. However, I think that colors are waves, and I wonder if black looks black because the waves cancel each other out and don't emit light. On the contrary, I wonder if white looks white because the waves are disturbed and emit light. That's how I interpret it.

ひかりのしるし
sign of light

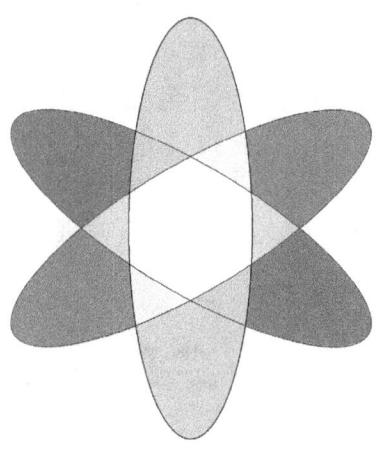

仮説 HYPOTHESIS

上昇気流(アセンション)体験や覚醒体験を経て思うこと
Thoughts after the Ascension Experience and the Awakening Experience

　誰にでも人には自己に内在する存在が存在していて、その存在に気が付かずに生活をしているのではないかと僕は仮説を立てています。

　I hypothesize that everyone has an inner existence within themselves, and that they live their lives without being aware of this existence.

　しかし、内的探求をすれば、自己に内在する存在を心の目で見ることが出来るようになっています。

　However, through inner inquiry, we are able to see with the mind's eye the presence within ourselves.

　その存在に気が付けた者だけが、その存在と繋(つな)がり、その存在と対話し、その存在の叡智(えいち)を授(さず)かり、その存在の教えを享受(きょうじゅ)して、その存在に意識が宿っている事実を知ります。

　Only those who become aware of that existence can connect with it, communicate with it, receive its wisdom, enjoy its teachings, and know the fact that consciousness dwells in that existence.

そして、その存在のアイデンティティ（存在証明）を夢のように共有することが出来るようになっています。そういった資質を人は持っています。

And it is possible to share the identity of that existence (existence proof) like a dream. People have those qualities.

しかし、外界の現実世界は取り留めなく過ぎて行くがゆえに、人間は外界の世界に対応する術を充分に身に付けています。結果、内的世界を忘れてしまっているのではないかと、考察しています。

However, because the real world of the outside world passes by haphazardly, humans are well equipped to deal with it. As a result, I am considering whether I have forgotten the inner world.

もしかしたら、幼少期は、こちらの内的世界の方が当然の世界だったのではないかとさえ思えてなりません。

I can't help but think that maybe this inner world was more natural in my childhood.

しかし、大人になって行く過程で、いつの間にかこのことを忘れてしまっている。そういった事実、現実があるのではないかと、考察しています。

However, in the process of becoming an adult, I forgot about this before I knew it. I believe that such a fact exists.

しかし、そのことに気が付けた人間は、上昇気流（アセンション）を体験し、覚醒体験まで教え導かれて行きます。
　However, humans who have noticed this experience an updraft (ascension) and are guided to an awakening experience.

　それが定（さだ）めと知って覚え書きのように書き示しておきます。あなた様に幸あれ。
　Knowing that this is the rule of this world, I write it down like a memorandum. good luck to you

当たり前のことかもしれないけどメモ
This may be a matter of course, but a note

　人と喋る時は、相手の顔を見ながら喋ること。
　When talking to someone, look at their face when you speak.

　相手を見ずに喋ると、なぜか、上手くいかなくなる。
　If you talk without looking at the other person, for some reason it will not go well.

　なんでだろう…
　I wonder why…

　相手の顔色を伺わないと相手に合わさずに一方的なお喋りになってしまうからだろうか、それとも、ネット空間と一緒で文字列的な会話になってしまって頭と頭で会話しているような表情のない脳内空間でのやりとりになってしまうからだろうか…
　Is it because if you don't ask the other person's complexion, you won't be in sync with the other person and the conversation will be one-sided? Or is it because, like the Internet space, the conversation becomes a string of characters, and it becomes an exchange in the brain space without facial expressions, like a conversation between thoughts…

　なんでそうなるのか、本当のところはよくわからないけど
　I don't really know why, but

とにかく、相手の様子を見ながら話をしたほうが、相手のシグナルが見えるからか、相手ありきで話が進むからか、いろいろ理由はあるだろうけれども、相手に集中して、相手の様子を見ながら話をしたほうが良い。
Anyway, it's better to talk while looking at the other person, so you can see the other person's signals, so the conversation progresses with the other person. There may be various reasons, but it is better to concentrate on the other person and talk while watching the situation of the other person.

その方が上手く行く。
It works better.

思想と思想のぶつかり合い
clash of ideas

　思想と思想のぶつかり合い、頭で動くとぶつかっちゃう。だけれども、心で動くとどうなるか、考えてみてほしい。
　Thoughts collide with each other, and if you move your head, they will collide. But think about what happens when you move with your mind.

　結論は後程…
　Conclusion later…

好きをトリガーにする
Trigger your favorite meter.

これ、好きぃっていうキッカケがはたらいた時だけ動く。
It works only when the trigger of "I like this" works.

これが、行動の第一原理。
This is the first principle of action.

それ以外は、もう何にも考えないんだ。
Other than that, I can't think of anything else.

どんなことでもね。
No matter what.

そうすれば、好きを道しるべにできる。
Then love will be your guide.

自己愛のすすめ
Advice on self-love

自己愛の利点。
Benefits of self-love.

自分を愛することができて初めて精神的自立が生まれます。
Only when you can love yourself do you become spiritually independent.

自分を愛するというのは、自分の体に滋養（じよう）を与えることになるんですね。
Loving yourself means nourishing your body.

自分の体にとって愛という栄養を受け取ることになります。
You will receive nourishment of love for your body.

この体にとって、これほど頼もしいことはないわけです。
There is nothing more reliable than this for my body.

健やかな感情も芽生えていきますし、健やかな感覚も得られてくることでしょう。そういった利点を得ることができます。
A healthy feeling will grow, and a healthy feeling will be obtained. You can get those benefits.

愛を与え、愛を受け取る、そういった循環（じゅんかん）、
Giving love and receiving love, such a cycle,

愛のループが生まれてくると、この体は喜びに満ちた状態となっていって心から嬉しく思うようになっていきます。
When the loop of love is born, this body will be in a joyful state and you will be happy from the bottom of your heart.

これを、続けていくと、精神的自立への道しるべとなっていって、あなた様を上昇へと導いていくことでしょう。
If you continue to do this, it will become a guidepost to your mental independence and will lead you to rise.

そう、それは、故（ゆえ）に、正（まさ）しく、あなた様の道しるべとなってまいりましょう。
Yes, that's exactly why it will be your guidepost.

思考の判断基準
Thinking Criteria

思考がネガティブだと、ハートに苦しみを感じます。
When your thoughts are negative, you feel pain in your heart.

思考がポジティブだと、ハートに心地良さを感じます。
When your thoughts are positive, you feel comfort in your heart.

もっとハッキリわかりやすい例を挙げますと、恋愛をしている時、好きな人のことを想うあまりにハートがキュンキュンして、居ても立っても居られなくなる経験は誰もがお持ちなのではないでしょうか。
To give a more clear and easy-to-understand example, when you are in love. I think everyone has had the experience of thinking about someone they love so much that their hearts pounded and they couldn't stand still.

それは、胸の中心、ハートの中心に、目では見えない何かが存在している証拠なのではないでしょうか。
I think it's proof that something invisible exists in the center of the chest, the center of the heart.

また、このことに気が付いてまいりますと、ハートの中心に意識を向けるようになっていきます。自然とハートの状態に目がいき、今、心地よい状態かなぁ、そうじゃないかなぁ、と、今、思考している内容が良いことか、はたまた悪いことかを瞬時に判断できるようになっていきます。
　Also, as you become aware of this, you will begin to turn your attention to the center of your heart. You will naturally observe the state of your heart. You will be able to instantly judge whether what you are thinking is good or bad, such as whether it is comfortable or not.

　心地よいと思えばそのまま進んで行けば良い訳ですし、心地よくないと感じるならば、その思考をやめれば良い訳です。
　If you think it's comfortable, you can go ahead as it is, If you feel uncomfortable, stop thinking about it.

　そういった判断基準となる指標に、言い変えるならば、目印になってくれているのではないでしょうか。
　To put it another way, they serve as indicators for such judgment criteria.

　ハートの中心にその人のコアとなる存在が潜んでいる可能性を感じます。
　I feel the possibility that the existence that becomes the core of that person is lurking in the center of the heart.

胸腺 THYMUS

　図書館で読んだ本の中で、これは、って思った情報がありましたので引用していきます。
　In the book I read at the library, there was information that I thought was this, so I'm going to quote it.

医学の書物です。
It's a medical book.

　まだ歴史が浅く、定説が確立しにくい分野である神経生理学においても、モントリオールにある臨床医学研究所のデーヴィッド・ホロビンが、免疫系の機能を円滑（えんかつ）に働かせるためには「プロスタグランジンE1」というホルモン様物質がひじょうに重要であると主張している。
　Even in neurophysiology, which has a short history and is difficult to establish an established theory, Dr. David Horobin of the Institute of Clinical Medicine in Montreal believes that a hormone called prostaglandin E1 is necessary for the smooth functioning of the immune system. claims that similar substances are very important.

　また、オックスフォード大学出身の科学者であるホロビンは、食事療法によって免疫系の調節、とくにがんを抑える、T細胞の調節ができることも強調している。

Horobin, a scientist from Oxford University, also emphasizes that diet can modulate the immune system, especially T cells, which fight cancer.

プロスタグランジンE1は、T細胞が成熟する場所である、胸腺（きょうせん）に大量に貯蔵されていることが知られている。
Prostaglandin E1 is known to be abundantly stored in the thymus, where T cells mature.

T細胞が欠如してB細胞が異常に活発なマウスをつくると、その個体はいずれ自己免疫疾患であるエリテマトーデス（SLE＝全身性紅斑性狼瘡｛ぜんしんせいこうはんせいろうそう｝）にかかったマウスと同じような死に方をする。
If you create mice that lack T cells and have hyperactive B cells, they eventually die in a manner similar to mice with the autoimmune disease lupus erythematosus (SLE).

ところがホロビンは、そのマウスにプロスタグランジンE1を与えるとT細胞が正常値に戻り、B細胞の活動も正常化して長生きするということを発見したのである。
Horobin, however, discovered that when prostaglandin E1 was given to the mice, T cells returned to normal levels and B cell activity normalized, leading to longer life.

【参考文献】内なる治癒力 こころと免疫をめぐる新しい医学 （著者）スティーヴン・ロック＋ダグラス・コリガン （監修）：池見酉次郎 （訳）田中彰＋堀雅明＋井上哲彰＋浦尾弥須子＋上野圭一

文章の意味はわからなくとも、胸の中心に重要な「プロスタグランジンE1」を大量に貯蔵する場所、胸腺（きょうせん）があることが観て取れます。

Even if you don't understand the meaning of the sentence, you can see that there is a place where a large amount of important "prostaglandin E1" is stored in the center of the chest, the thymus.

　読みながら首を縦（たて）に振りながら、「ふ〜ん」って思ってました。また、この本では、最後の締めくくりにこんなことが書かれています。

Shaking my head while reading, I thought, "Hmm." Also, at the end of the book, it says:

　デーヴィッド・マクレーランドが「マザー・テレサ効果」と命名した、治療にまつわる魅力的な現象である。

It's a fascinating therapeutic phenomenon that David McClelland has dubbed the "Mother Teresa Effect."

　マザー・テレサは生涯をカルカッタの貧民救済に捧げたノーベル平和賞の受賞者だが、マクレーランドは学生たちに彼女の仕事ぶりを描いた感動的な映画を見せ、その前後に採取した血液像に変化があることに興味をそそられた。

Mother Teresa is a Nobel Peace Prize laureate who dedicated her life to helping the poor of Calcutta. McClelland showed her students a moving film depicting her work, and was intrigued by the changes in her blood drawn before and after.

映画を観たあとの学生たちの免疫グロブリンの数値が、わずかだが上昇し、免疫系の機能が向上したことがわかったからである。

After watching the movie, the students' immunoglobulin levels rose slightly, suggesting that their immune systems functioned better.

その後、彼はさまざまな方法でこの「マザー・テレサ効果」を確認した。映画を見せる代わりに、大学院生たちに次の二つのことについて深く考えるように指示したこともある。

Later, he confirmed this "Mother Teresa effect" in various ways. Instead of showing the film, he once asked graduate students to ponder two things.

すなわち、それまでの人生で「自分が誰かに深く愛されたとき」と「自分が誰かを愛したとき」のことをよく考えさせたのだ。やはり効果はあった。

In other words, it made me think about "when I was deeply loved by someone" and "when I loved someone" in my life. After all, it was effective.

マクレーランドはじつは前から体験的にそのことを知っていて、効果があることを信じてもいたのである。

In fact, McClelland had known about it experientially for a long time, and believed that it worked.

「風邪をひいたときなど、わたしはよく、愛した人のことや愛された人のことを考えるんです。それだけで、風邪が治ってしまったことも二、三度ありますよ。絶対に効くというわけじゃありませんがね。いくらやってもダメで、風邪がひどくなった時もありました。しかし、役に立ちます。」

When I catch a cold, I think about the times when I loved and when I was loved. There have been two or three times when I've gotten over my cold just by doing that. That doesn't mean it will work for sure. No matter how much I tried, it didn't work, and there was a time when I had a bad cold. But it helps.

愛がもつ力に対するマクレーランドの強い信念は、彼が擁護(ようご)する現代医学に大きな示唆(しさ)を与えている。

McClelland's strong belief in the power of love has great implications for the modern medicine he advocates.

人間の精神に備わったこの貴重な力は、これまで見すごされてきたが、彼にいわせれば、それこそが治療という現象における内的な原動力なのである。

This precious power of the human mind has hitherto been overlooked. But, according to him, that is the inner driving force in the phenomenon of therapy.

「病院の環境を変えることによって、いろいろなことができます」マクレーランドはあるとき、医学関係者の集まりでこんな発言をした。

"By changing the hospital environment, we can do many things." McClelland once said at a meeting of medical professionals:

「病院をリラックスできる場に、自然に思いやりのこころが生まれるような場に、たえず何かに追われているような気分から解放されるような場にすればいいんです。

We need to make the hospital a place where people can relax, a place where compassion naturally arises, a place where they are freed from the constant feeling of being chased by something.

つまり、健康な環境にすればね。医師も看護師もソーシャルワーカーも、その気になればできますよ。だれかを愛することは、愛する相手の健康にとってひじょうにいい効果があるんです。そして、たぶん、愛した人自身の健康にとっても」

In other words, in a healthy environment. Doctors, nurses, and social workers can do it if they want to. Loving someone is very good for the health of the person you love. And, perhaps, you can expect an effect on the health of the loved one himself.

【参考文献】内なる治癒力 こころと免疫をめぐる新しい医学
（著者）スティーヴン・ロック＋ダグラス・コリガン
（監修）：池見酉次郎（訳）田中彰＋堀雅明＋井上哲彰＋浦尾弥須子＋上野圭一

これを読みながら、私が、推奨する愛と友情のエネルギーの使い方が読んで字の如（ごと）く証明されているかのような錯覚（さっかく）に陥（おちい）りました。

As I read this, I had the illusion that the use of love and friendship energy I was recommending was literally proven.

　もし、愛と友情のエネルギーの使い方を実践することによって、胸腺（きょうせん）に刺激が与えられ、T細胞を強力に活性化する事象を確認することさえできれば、医学的にがんを抑える効果があると証明されたことになります。

If we can confirm that the thymus is stimulated by practicing how to use the energy of love and friendship and strongly activates T cells, we can say that it is medically effective in suppressing cancer.

　と、まぁ、そういうことを思いついたわけです。しかし、医学者でもなく、科学者でもない、わたしが、これを確認するには、どうすればいいのだろう…今、すぐに、答えが見つからなかったため、保留して次に進みます。

And, well, that's what I came up with. But I am neither a medical doctor nor a scientist, how can I confirm this? Right now, I haven't found an answer, so I'll put it on hold and move on.

T細胞（T cells）

　胸腺（きょうせん）の調査で、T細胞を活性化できれば、免疫機能がアップしてがんを抑制（よくせい）することができるという話でした。今回は、それに引き続きT細胞とはなにかを調査しました。僕の言葉で書いても、説得力が欠けるため、本の中身を引用します。

　In the thymus investigation, I was told that if T cells can be activated, the immune function can be improved and cancer can be suppressed. This time, we continued to investigate what T cells are. Even if I write it in my own words, it lacks persuasiveness, so I will quote the contents of the book.

　　免疫機能が、がん細胞を攻撃する仕組みが次第にわかってきています。
　　The mechanism by which the immune system attacks cancer cells is gradually being understood.

　　ひとつが、ナチュラル・キラー（NK）細胞によるものです。NK細胞は、原始的な本能をもっていて、自分ではないものを見つけると即刻、攻撃を仕掛け、排除しようとします。ひじょうに強力な殺傷力があるので、活性化させることでがんが劇的に縮小したという例はたくさん出ています。
　　One is by natural killer (NK) cells. NK cells have a primitive instinct, and as soon as they find something they are not, they attack and try to eliminate it. It has a very strong killing power, so there are many cases

where cancers have shrunk dramatically by activating it.

NK細胞は、組織的に管理されて動くのではなく、ゲリラ的に神出鬼没といった行動を得意としています。
NK cells are good at acting in a guerilla-like manner, rather than being systematically controlled.

もうひとつが、T細胞（ヘルパーT細胞、キラーT細胞、サプレッサーT細胞）を中心としたシステマチックな免疫活動があります。
Another is systematic immune activity centered on T cells (helper T cells, killer T cells, suppressor T cells).

T細胞は、抗原抗体反応とよく似た抗原・T細胞受容体反応に支配されていますから、抗原を認識するという過程が、必要です。T細胞は、すぐそばにがん細胞があったとしても、抗原として認識できなければ見逃してしまいます。
Since T cells are governed by antigen-T cell receptor reactions that are very similar to antigen-antibody reactions, the process of recognizing antigens is necessary. Even if there are cancer cells nearby, T cells will miss them if they cannot recognize them as antigens.

抗原があることをT細胞に知らせるのが、抗原提示細胞と呼ばれるマクロファージや樹状（じゅじょう）細胞です。抗原提示細胞は、がん細胞を取り込んで消化し、その情報をヘルパーT細胞に伝えます。

Macrophages and dendritic cells called antigen-presenting cells inform T cells of the presence of antigens. Antigen-presenting cells ingest and digest cancer cells and pass on the information to helper T cells.

情報を受けたヘルパーT細胞はサイトカイン類を放出することで、がん細胞を攻撃するキラーT細胞に抗原を作らせ、活性化させてがん細胞排除の体制を作るのです。
The helper T cells that receive the information release cytokines to make the killer T cells that attack cancer cells produce antigens and activate them to create a system to eliminate cancer cells.

【参考文献】がんを治す医療辞典決定版　最新の現代医学から確かな代替療法まで。
「がん」と闘うための総合辞典
（総監修）帯津良一

　読みながら、縦（たて）に首を振りながら「ふ〜ん」って思いました。
Shaking my head while reading, I thought, "Hmm."

　複雑な仕組みでがんを抑制する機能が人間に備わっているんだなぁと感心するのでした。
I was impressed that humans have the ability to suppress cancer through a complex mechanism.

　話の中身がわからなくとも、独自に動くナチュラル・キラー（NK）細胞と、システマチックに動くT細胞達が、体の免疫機能を担っていることが、なんとなしに理解できてたらいいのかなぁと思いました。

Even if you don't understand the content of the story, it would be nice if you could somehow understand that natural killer (NK) cells that move independently and T cells that move systematically are responsible for the body's immune function.

もちろん、読み込んで理解もしておりますが、おさらいの意味を込めて記述していきます。
Of course, I have read and understood it, but I will write it with the meaning of a review.

システマチックに動くT細胞達の説明をしますと、キラーT細胞と言うのが、がん細胞を攻撃する役目を担っていて、抗原提示細胞（マクロファージや樹状細胞）が、がんを発見し、がんを認知して、がん細胞を取り込み、その情報をヘルパーT細胞に伝えて、ヘルパーT細胞がサイトカイン類を放出してキラーT細胞に抗原を提示し、キラーT細胞を活性化させ、攻撃態勢を整えてから、がん細胞を攻撃する、システマチックな仕組みをT細胞達はもっています。
To explain T cells that move systematically, killer T cells play a role in attacking cancer cells, and antigen-presenting cells (macrophages and dendritic cells) discover cancer. Then, it recognizes cancer, takes in cancer cells, conveys the information to helper T cells, and helper T cells release cytokines, present antigens to killer T cells, and activate killer T cells. T cells have a systematic mechanism to attack cancer cells after preparing to attack them.

人体にある細胞達が連携して、人間の免疫機能を担っている事象が本を読みながら見えてきました。

　As I read the book, I began to see how the cells in the human body work together to support the human immune system.

免疫細胞の種類の整理
types of immune cells

免疫細胞の種類の整理をしておきたいと思います。
I would like to organize the types of immune cells.

これまでに、T細胞達が免疫機能に活躍していることを書いてきました、が、しかし、T細胞達とは何かといったことについて、言及をしてきませんでした。ここでは、その部分を紐解（ひもと）いていきたいと思います。
So far, I have written that T cells are active in immune function, but I have not mentioned what T cells are. I would like to break down that part here.

人間の血液は、赤血球、白血球、血小板と液体成分の血しょうで成り立っていると学生の頃に理科か化学で習った記憶がある方が多いのではないかと想像しています。その中の、白血球のお話です。
I imagine that there are many people who remember that human blood is made up of red blood cells, white blood cells, platelets, and plasma, a liquid component, that they learned in science or chemistry when they were students. This is the story of the white blood cells in it.

白血球には、リンパ球、単球（マクロファージ、樹状細胞）、顆粒球（かりゅうきゅう）が含まれています。その中のリンパ球には、Tリンパ球、Bリンパ球、ナチュラル・キラー（NK）細胞が含まれています。その中のTリンパ球には、キラーT細胞やヘルパーT細胞が含まれています。
　Leukocytes include lymphocytes, monocytes (macrophages, dendritic cells), and granulocytes. Lymphocytes in it include T lymphocytes, B lymphocytes, and natural killer (NK) cells. Among the T lymphocytes are killer T cells and helper T cells.

　ここまで、読んでいただければ、これまで、説明してきた、T細胞はTリンパ球と呼ばれていることに気がつきます。胸腺から出てくるのはTリンパ球（T細胞）なんだなぁと認識できれば御の字です。
　If you have read this far, you will notice that the T cells that we have explained so far are called T lymphocytes. If you can recognize that it is T lymphocytes (T cells) that come out of the thymus, you are in luck.

ヘルパーT細胞とサイトカイン
Helper T cells and cytokines

ヘルパーT細胞が出すサイトカインの説明を引用します。
I will quote the description of cytokines produced by helper T cells.

　サイトカインは、一つひとつの細胞から分泌されるタンパク質で、細胞間伝達分子と呼ばれているように、様々な情報を運び、その情報によって細胞を活性化させたり、鎮（しず）めたりする役割を果たしています。
　Cytokines are proteins secreted from each cell, and as they are called intercellular communication molecules, carry various information and play the role of activating or calming cells according to the information.

　構造や作用によって、いくつもの種類のサイトカインがあることがわかっています。がん細胞と免疫にかんするサイトカインとしては、インターロイキン、インターフェロン、腫瘍壊死因子（しゅようえしいんし）がよく知られています。
　We know that there are several types of cytokines, depending on their structure and action. Interleukins, interferons, and tumor necrosis factors are well-known cytokines related to cancer cells and immunity.

がん細胞が発見されると、マクロファージや樹状細胞が、がん細胞やその死骸を食べると同時に、どんな種類のがんが発生したのかをT細胞に知らせます。情報を受けたT細胞は興奮し活性化されます。そして、ヘルパーT細胞が、攻撃部隊であるキラーT細胞を目覚めさせ、がん細胞に攻撃を仕掛けるのです。

When cancer cells are found, macrophages and dendritic cells eat the cancer cells and their dead bodies, and at the same time, tell T cells what kind of cancer has developed. Upon receiving the information, the T cells are excited and activated. The helper T cells awaken the attacking force, the killer T cells, and attack the cancer cells.

　この一連のシステムの仲立ちをしているのが、サイトカインです。IL-2、IL-12などが刺激伝達の役割を果たします。免疫細胞のひじょうに緻密（ちみつ）なシステムがよく言われますが、サイトカインがあってはじめて成り立っているものなのです。

Cytokines mediate this series of systems. IL-2, IL-12, etc. play a role in stimulus transmission. It is often said that immune cells are a very well-developed and elaborate system, but it is precisely because of cytokines that this system is able to function well.

【参考文献】がんを治す医療辞典決定版　最新の現代医学から確かな代替療法まで。「がん」と闘うための総合辞典
（総監修）帯津良一

ヘルパーT細胞の説明を引用します。
I will quote the description of helper T cells.

　免疫の研究が進んで、興味深い事実が数多くわかってきました。その一つが、免疫には「液性免疫」と「細胞性免疫」があるということです。
Advances in immunological research have revealed many interesting facts. One of them is that there are "humoral immunity" and "cellular immunity" in immunity.

　液性免疫は、真菌や細菌に対する免疫です。マクロファージや樹状細胞が真菌や細菌を取り込み、その情報をヘルパーT細胞に伝えます。ヘルパーT細胞は二種類あり、この時に活性化するのは、２型のヘルパーT細胞（Th2）です。Th2は、IL-4、IL-5、IL-10などを分泌して、B細胞などを刺激します。
"Humoral immunity" is immunity against fungi and bacteria. Macrophages and dendritic cells take up fungi and bacteria and pass on the information to helper T cells. There are two types of helper T cells, and type 2 helper T cells (Th2) are activated at this time. Th2 secretes IL-4, IL-5, IL-10, etc. to stimulate B cells and others.

細胞性免疫は、がん細胞などに対する免疫です。マクロファージや樹状細胞は、がん細胞を取り込んだのち、1型ヘルパーT細胞（Th1）を活性化させるためのサイトカインであるIL-12を放出します。Th1は、IL-2やインターフェロンγ（IFN-γ）を出して、キラーT細胞やNK細胞を活性化させます。

Cell-mediated immunity is immunity against cancer cells. After engulfing cancer cells, macrophages and dendritic cells release IL-12, a cytokine that activates type 1 helper T cells (Th1). Th1 secretes IL-2 and interferon-γ (IFN-γ) to activate killer T cells and NK cells.

　液性免疫と細胞性免疫は、お互いに微妙なバランスを取り合っています。2つの細胞には、一方が高まりすぎると、一方を抑制してしまうという関係があることがわかってきました。

Humoral and cellular immunity are in a delicate balance with each other. It has been found that there is a relationship between the two cells, in which if one is too high, the other is suppressed.

　つまり、がん細胞を攻撃する細胞性免疫が十分に働くためには、液性免疫の作用が抑えられなければならないのです。

In other words, in order for cell-mediated immunity, which attacks cancer cells, to work sufficiently, the action of humoral immunity must be suppressed.

免疫力は、「液性」「細胞性」を区別することなく全体で「高まる」「低下する」という図式で語られてきましたが、より深く研究していくと、デリケートなバランスがあることがわかってきたのです。
Immunity has been described in terms of "increase" and "decrease" as a whole without distinguishing between "humoral" and "cellular". However, upon deeper study, it became clear that there is a delicate balance.

免疫が高まるといっても、がんを治療するには、細胞性免疫の方を高めないと意味がないということになります。
In order to treat cancer, it is meaningless unless cell-mediated immunity is enhanced.

そのためには、IL-12やIFN-γというサイトカインの産生で促（うなが）すことが必要となってくるのです。
For that purpose, it is necessary to promote the production of cytokines such as IL-12 and IFN-γ.

【参考文献】がんを治す医療辞典決定版　最新の現代医学から確かな代替療法まで。「がん」と闘うための総合辞典
（総監修）帯津良一

読みながら、首を縦（たて）に振りながら「ふ～ん」って思いました。
Shaking my head while reading, I thought, "Hmm."

専門用語を見ると、読み込む前に「うっ」となって敬遠（けいえん）してしまいがちですが、言っていることは単純で、私達の人体は、真菌や細菌の病気に対しては、２型のヘルパーT細胞を介してB細胞などを刺激して液性免疫を獲得（かくとく）しています。
　When you see technical terms, you tend to shy away from them before reading them, but what they are saying is simple. Our human body acquires humoral immunity against fungal and bacterial diseases by stimulating B cells via type 2 helper T cells.

　また、がん細胞やウィルスに感染した細胞（コロナや風邪）の病気に対しては、１型のヘルパーT細胞を介してキラーT細胞やNK細胞を活性化させて細胞性免疫を獲得（かくとく）しています。
　In addition, against diseases caused by cancer cells and virus-infected cells (coronavirus and colds), cell-mediated immunity is acquired by activating killer T cells and NK cells via type 1 helper T cells.

　この２つの免疫機能は絶妙なバランスを保ちながら作用していて、どちらか一方が高まれば、どちらか一方が抑えられる仕組みとなっています。
　These two immune functions work while maintaining a perfect balance, and if one increases, the other is suppressed.

　このことから、分かってくることは、T細胞が中心になって免疫系を支配していることが見えてきます。

What we can see from this is that T cells play a central role in controlling the immune system.

ここが肝心なところと理解していただけたら御の字です。
I hope you can understand that this is the key point.

T細胞は胸腺から作られていることが知られていますから、T細胞を安定的に供給できるように胸腺を活性化することができれば、真菌や細菌の病気も、がんやウィルスに感染した細胞の病気（コロナや風邪）も、バランス良く免疫を獲得（かくとく）することが可能になると推測できます。
It is known that T cells are made from the thymus. If the thymus can be activated and a stable supply of T cells can be obtained, it will be possible to acquire well-balanced immunity against fungal and bacterial diseases, as well as cancer and virus-infected cell diseases (coronavirus and colds). We can assume that it will be possible.

がんもコロナも、ほとんどの病気が胸腺から発生するT細胞にかかっていることが見えてきます。胸腺を活性化することさえできれば、怖いものなしとなることが手に取るように推測できるわけです。
We can see that cancer, corona, and most diseases depend on the work of T cells generated from the thymus. As long as you can activate the thymus, you can guess that there will be nothing to fear.

自律神経
Autonomic nerves

　自律神経を主軸に免疫機能を調べました。その内容を引用します。
　We investigated the immune function centering on the autonomic nervous system. I will quote its contents.

　自律神経は本来、心臓や胃腸、呼吸器、血管、汗腺などのはたらきをコントロールしている神経です。脳の指令を受けずに独立してはたらくことから、自律神経と呼ばれています。脳が休んでいる睡眠時間でも、自律神経のコントロールによって心臓は休まずにはたらき続けています。
　Autonomic nerves are originally nerves that control the functions of the heart, gastrointestinal tract, respiratory system, blood vessels, and sweat glands. It is called the autonomic nervous system because it works independently without receiving commands from the brain. Even during sleep, when the brain is resting, the heart continues to work without rest due to the control of the autonomic nervous system.

　自律神経には、交感神経と副交感神経があり、正反対のはたらきをしています。交感神経は運動や緊張をしたときなどに優位になり、心臓の拍動を高め、血管を収縮させ、体を活動的な状態にします。

The autonomic nervous system consists of the sympathetic and parasympathetic nervous systems, which have opposite functions. The sympathetic nervous system becomes dominant during exercise and tension, increasing the heartbeat, constricting blood vessels, and putting the body into an active state.

　一方の副交感神経は、休息しているときに優位になる神経で、心拍数を下げ、血管を拡張します。副交感神経がはたらくことで、心身がリラックスし、消化液の分泌や排便が促（うなが）されます。
The parasympathetic nerves, on the other hand, are dominant at rest, slowing the heart rate and dilating blood vessels. By working the parasympathetic nerves, the mind and body are relaxed, and the secretion of digestive juices and defecation are urged.

　白血球は、赤血球とともに血液の重要な成分のひとつです。赤血球が栄養分や酸素を細胞に運び、老廃物や二酸化炭素を回収するという仕事をしています。
White blood cells are one of the important components of blood along with red blood cells. Red blood cells carry nutrients and oxygen to cells and remove waste products and carbon dioxide.

　一方、白血球は感染やがんから体を守るはたらきをしています。その数は、赤血球が１０００個に対して白血球が１個という割合です。

On the other hand, white blood cells work to protect the body from infection and cancer. The ratio is 1 white blood cell to 1000 red blood cells.

白血球の中身を見ると、健康な人では顆粒球(かりゅうきゅう)がおおむね6割に対して、リンパ球がおおむね4割の割合です。

Looking at the contents of white blood cells, in a healthy person, about 60% are granulocytes and about 40% are lymphocytes.

顆粒球は、真菌や大腸菌、細胞の死骸、カビなどの比較的大きなサイズの異物を食べて処理します。このときに、酸化力の強い物質(活性酸素)を出して異物を破壊します。活性酸素ががんの発生、増殖と大いにかかわっています。

Granulocytes eat and process relatively large-sized foreign substances such as fungi, E. coli, dead cells, and molds. At this time, substances with strong oxidizing power (active oxygen) are released to destroy foreign substances. Active oxygen is greatly involved in the development and growth of cancer.

リンパ球は、ウィルスなど小さな異物を排除するときに活躍します。リンパ球は、異物を「抗原」として認識すると、「抗体」と呼ばれるタンパク質を作り、異物に対して無毒化するようにはたらきかけます。リンパ球には、ナチュラル・キラー(NK)細胞、T細胞、B細胞などの種類があります。

Lymphocytes are active in eliminating small foreign substances such as viruses. When lymphocytes recognize foreign substances as "antigens", they produce proteins called "antibodies" and work to detoxify the foreign substances. Types of lymphocytes include natural killer (NK) cells, T cells, and B cells.

　自律神経と白血球の間には、緊密な関係があります。
　There is a close relationship between autonomic nerves and white blood cells.

　自律神経は、内臓のはたらきを調整するときに神経の末端から神経伝達物質を分泌します。交感神経からはアドレナリンが、副交感神経からはアセチルコリンが出て内臓に緊張やリラックスの指令を出すのです。
　Autonomic nerves secrete neurotransmitters from nerve endings to regulate the function of internal organs. Adrenaline is released from the sympathetic nerves, and acetylcholine is released from the parasympathetic nerves, which give commands to the internal organs to induce tension and relaxation.

　アドレナリンは、心も体も緊張させます。心臓の鼓動を上げ、血管を収縮させます。逆に、アセチルコリンは、心身をリラックスさせます。消化や吸収、排泄を促進する作用もあります。
　Adrenaline makes the mind and body tense. Increases heart rate and constricts blood vessels. Conversely, acetylcholine relaxes the mind and body. It also promotes digestion, absorption and excretion.

白血球の顆粒球とリンパ球では、アドレナリンやアセチルコリンに対して違う反応をします。顆粒球はアドレナリンで活発になり、アセチルコリンで活動が抑制されます。リンパ球はその反対です。

White blood cells, granulocytes and lymphocytes, respond differently to adrenaline and acetylcholine. Granulocytes are activated by adrenaline and inhibited by acetylcholine. Lymphocytes are the opposite.

　つまり、交感神経が緊張すると、アドレナリンが分泌され顆粒球が反応します。副交感神経が優位になると、アセチルコリンが分泌されてリンパ球が反応します。反応するとは、活性化し、数も増えるということを意味しています。

In other words, when the sympathetic nerves become tense, adrenaline is secreted and granulocytes respond. When the parasympathetic nerve becomes dominant, acetylcholine is secreted and lymphocytes respond. To react means to activate and increase in number.

　顆粒球は、外から侵入してきた比較的大きな異物を攻撃する細胞です。つかまえて溶かしてしまう攻撃パターンをもっていますが、このときに武器として使うのが活性酸素です。

Granulocytes are cells that attack relatively large foreign substances that have invaded from the outside. It has an attack pattern that catches and melts, but it uses active oxygen as a weapon at this time.

活性酸素はひじょうに不安定な酸素のことで、安定するために周りの分子から電子を奪い取ります。電子が奪われた分子は、酸化という現象を起こし、一気に活性を失ってしまいます。さびてボロボロになってしまうのです。この性質を利用して、顆粒球は異物を処理しています。

Reactive oxygen is oxygen that is so unstable that it steals electrons from surrounding molecules in order to stabilize it. Molecules from which electrons have been deprived undergo a phenomenon called oxidation, and lose their activity all at once. It will rust and fall apart. Using this property, granulocytes process foreign substances.

　交感神経が緊張して顆粒球が多くなると、活性酸素の量も増えてきます。

When the sympathetic nervous system becomes tense and the number of granulocytes increases, the amount of active oxygen also increases.

　通常、活性酸素は酵素によって除去されますが、酵素の能力を超えて発生した活性酸素は、あたりかまわず攻撃を仕掛けます。細胞が酸化し、DNAも傷つけられます。そのことが、細胞のがん化につながります。がん細胞が増殖していく原因にもなっているのです。

Normally, active oxygen is removed by enzymes, but active oxygen generated beyond the ability of enzymes will attack regardless of the surroundings. Cells are oxidized and DNA is damaged. This leads to cell carcinogenesis. It also causes cancer cells to grow.

活性酸素は、呼吸や細胞の新陳代謝によっても発生しますが、顆粒球が発するものがかなりの割合を占めるといわれています。つまり、顆粒球が増えれば増えるほど、がんは発生しやすくなります。

Active oxygen is also generated by respiration and cell metabolism. However, it is said that active oxygen emitted by granulocytes accounts for a considerable proportion. In other words, the more granulocytes there are, the more likely cancer is to develop.

がん治療のためには、顆粒球を増やさないようにしたほうがいいということになります。顆粒球が増えるということは、相対的にリンパ球が減ることを意味します。

For cancer treatment, it is better not to increase granulocytes. An increase in granulocytes means a relative decrease in lymphocytes.

顆粒球が増えることで、活性酸素による細胞のがん化が進み、がん細胞を排除するリンパ球の減少によって免疫力が下がるのですから、がん細胞にとっては最高に生きやすい環境といってもいいでしょう。

As granulocytes increase, cells become cancerous due to active oxygen, and as lymphocytes, which eliminate cancer cells, decrease, immunity weakens. Therefore, it can be said that it is the best environment for cancer cells to live.

つまり、がんを治すには、活性酸素を発生させる顆粒球を

少なくし、がんを排除しようとはたらくリンパ球を増やし、がん細胞が生きにくい環境を作ればいいわけです。

In other words, in order to cure cancer, it is necessary to reduce the number of granulocytes that generate active oxygen and increase the number of lymphocytes that try to eliminate cancer, thereby creating an environment in which cancer cells cannot survive.

がんを引き起こす要因。
Factors that cause cancer.

・はたらきすぎの寝不足さん
・Overworked and lack of sleep

睡眠をしっかりとれている場合は良いのですが、3〜4時間の睡眠で、はたらき続けている人は、顆粒球の数が異常に多くなってしまい、活性酸素の量も増え、細胞の酸化が進みます。注意が必要です。

It is good if you are getting enough sleep, but if you are working continuously with 3 to 4 hours of sleep, the number of granulocytes will increase abnormally, the amount of active oxygen will increase, and the cells will be oxidized.

・心の悩み
・Trouble of heart

　不安や悩みや悲しみといったストレスは、脳の大脳辺緑系で感知され、視床下部へ伝えられます。
　Stress such as anxiety, worry, and sadness is sensed in the brain's limbic system and transmitted to the hypothalamus.

　視床下部は、自律神経や内分泌などのコントロールを司る場所です。視床下部は、ストレス刺激を受けて、アドレナリンやノルアドレナリンを分泌させ、交感神経の緊張状態を作り出します。
　The hypothalamus is a place that controls the autonomic nervous system and endocrine. When the hypothalamus receives a stress stimulus, it secretes adrenaline and noradrenaline, creating a state of sympathetic nervous tension.

　その結果、心拍や呼吸が早まり、血圧が上がります。不安なことがあると、心拍が速くなるという体験はどなたにもあるのではないでしょうか。
　As a result, your heart rate and breathing speed up, and your blood pressure rises. We all know that anxiety makes your heart beat faster.

　顆粒球を増やし、リンパ球を減らし、血流を悪くさせるという、がんを発生させ、増殖させる環境をもたらすのです。

By increasing the number of granulocytes, decreasing the number of lymphocytes, and impairing blood flow, it creates an environment for cancer to develop and proliferate.

がん細胞の増殖を抑制し、治療にもって行くためには、リンパ球を増やして免疫力を上げなければなりません。
In order to suppress the growth of cancer cells and bring them to treatment, it is necessary to increase lymphocytes and boost immunity.

リンパ球は副交感神経を優位にすることで増やすことができます。
Lymphocytes can be increased by making the parasympathetic nerves dominant.

【参考文献】がんを治す医療辞典決定版　最新の現代医学から確かな代替療法まで。「がん」と闘うための総合辞典
（総監修）帯津良一

顆粒球（かりゅうきゅう）とは
What is a granulocyte?

細胞の中に殺菌作用のある成分を含んだ「顆粒」を持つ白血球の総称です。好中球、好酸球、塩基球の3種類に分けられます。
It is a general term for white blood cells that have "granules" containing components with bactericidal action in the cells. They are divided into three types: neutrophils, eosinophils, and basophils.

【参考文献】国立研究開発法人国立がん研究センターのホームページ

読みながら、首を縦（たて）に振りながら「ふ～ん」て思いました。
Shaking my head while reading, I thought, "Hmm."

　交感神経も副交感神経も、２種類のヘルパーＴ細胞と同様にお互いのバランスをとりながら作用し合っているんだなぁと思えたらいいのかなと思いました。
I thought it would be nice to think that the sympathetic nerves and parasympathetic nerves work together while balancing each other, just like two types of helper T cells.

　おそらく、どちらも必要で、バランスよく生活することが求められていると私は解釈しました。昼間は交感神経優位の状態で活動して、夜間は副交感神経を優位にして睡眠することを心がければバランスが良い生活サイクルになるのではないかと思います。
Perhaps both are necessary, and I interpret that we are required to live in a balanced manner. I think that if you try to sleep with the sympathetic nervous system dominant during the day and sleep with the parasympathetic nervous system dominant at night, you will have a well-balanced life cycle.

　と、ここまででしたら、今までの、調査と変わりがなかったのですが、ついに、見つけました。どうすれば、免疫力が上がったと証拠として提示できるのか、いわば判断できる、

評価対象物とは何か、その数値データはどうすれば得られるのか。その判断基準が見えてきました。

Finally, I found it. How can I show that my immunity has increased? In other words, what is the object of evaluation that can be judged? How can I get the numerical data? I found the criteria for that.

自律神経免疫療法の評価基準。
Evaluation criteria for autonomic nervous system immunotherapy.

治療はリンパ球の数や白血球のなかに占める割合をチェックして、効果を確認しながら進められます。
Treatment is carried out while confirming the effect by checking the number of lymphocytes and the percentage of white blood cells.

健康な人の場合、血液１mm^3（立方ミリメートル）あたり２３００〜２６００個くらいのリンパ球が含まれています。
In the case of a healthy person, 1 mm^3 (cubic millimeter) of blood contains about 2300 to 2600 lymphocytes.

２０００個くらいが下限で、これ以下になると免疫力が低下して病気になりやすくなると言われています。
About 2,000 is the lower limit, and it is said that if the number is less than this, the immune system will be weakened and people will become more susceptible to illness.

がん患者は１５００個でも相当いいほうです。１５００個以下、抗がん剤などの治療を受けていると１０００個程度、それ以下になっている場合もあるといいます。
　For cancer patients, 1500 is quite good. 1500 or less. It is said that there are cases where it is about 1000, or even less, when receiving treatment such as anticancer drugs.

　自律神経免疫療法では、リンパ球を２０００個程度にまで回復させるのが目標です。２０００個を超えてくると免疫力がじわじわと力をつけてくるのです。
　The goal of autonomic nervous system immunotherapy is to restore the number of lymphocytes to about 2000. When it exceeds 2000, the immune force gradually gains strength.

【参考文献】がんを治す医療辞典決定版　最新の現代医学から確かな代替療法まで。
「がん」と闘うための総合辞典
（総監修）帯津良一

　これが欲しかった。これです。私が調べたかったこと。
　I wanted this. This. what i wanted to find out.

　これを軸に愛と友情のエネルギーの使い方の評価をしていけばいいんだなってことがわかりました。
　I realized that I should evaluate how to use the energy of love and friendship based on this.

これをお読みの読者で、身近にがん患者様がいる場合、早急に愛と友情のエネルギーの使い方を試してみる価値がございます。
　If you are reading this and have a cancer patient close to you, Teach them how to use the energy of love and friendship as soon as possible. Worth a try.

　私は、これから、私なりの研究を進めていきたいと考えております。
　From now on, I would like to proceed with my own research.

　が、しかし、今すぐ結果が出せるものでもございません。
　However, it is not something that can produce results right away.

　臨床試験と呼ばれる類のものをクリアしなければ医学的に認められたことにならないからです。
　This is because it is not medically recognized unless it clears what is called a clinical trial.

　ですから、一朝一夕で達成できるようなものではございません。
　Therefore, it is not something that can be achieved overnight.

胸腺（きょうせん）のまとめ
Summary of Thymus

　愛と友情のエネルギーの使い方に医学的根拠はあるのか、その問いに答えると、愛の力により免疫機能への効果を期待する声が医学者の中から現れてきている事実を鑑（かんが）みても、人間の免疫機能を司る主要器官である胸腺がハートの中心あたりに潜んでいる事実を鑑（かんが）みても、これからの研究の余地があると結論づけます。

　Is there a medical basis for using the energy of love and friendship? I will answer that question. There is a fact that some medical scientists are expecting the effect of the power of love on the immune system. There is a fact that the thymus, the main organ that controls human immune function, is hidden in the heart. We conclude that there is room for further research.

　また。未解決の問題として愛と友情のエネルギーの使い方をすることにより医学的に胸腺に刺激が与えられ、免疫機能を司るT細胞などに影響を与え、人間の免疫機能がアップする事象の確認と証明がされていない事実がございます。

　Also, there is an open issue. At present, there is no evidence that using the energy of love and friendship can medically stimulate the thymus gland, affect T cells that control immune function, and improve human immune function.

今後の課題として、愛と友情のエネルギーの使い方をする前とした後の血液を採取して免疫機能にどれだけの影響が現れて、どれだけの効果が得られるのか、また、継続的に半年間、３年間と、愛と友情のエネルギーの使い方をした場合の結果をみて、どれだけの影響が現れて、どれだけの効果が得られるのか、調査できれば、医学的に免疫力を高める手法として証明されることになるのではないかと期待しています。

As a future task, I think that we will be able to see how much the immune function will be affected by collecting blood before and after using the energy of love and friendship, and how much effect will be obtained. In addition, you will be evaluated by looking at the results of using the energy of love and friendship continuously for 6 months to 3 years. If we can investigate how much influence appears and how much effect can be obtained, I hope that it will be proven as a method of improving immunity medically.

期待通りの結果が得られますと既存治療法などと併用して、がん治療に活かせる可能性を秘めているのではないかと推論づけています。

If the expected results can be obtained, it is speculated that there is a hidden possibility that it can be used in cancer treatment in combination with existing treatment methods.

もし、愛と友情のエネルギーの使い方に医学的なエビデンスや、科学的なエビデンスがあることが証明されてまいりますと、福島県でがんに怯（おび）えながら暮らしている人々の不安を少しでも軽減することが出来るようになるのではないかと期待して、この文書を締めくくらせていただきたいと思います。

　If it is proved that there is medical evidence and scientific evidence on how to use the energy of love and friendship, it will be possible to reduce the anxiety of people living in Fukushima Prefecture who are afraid of cancer. I hope it will be possible.

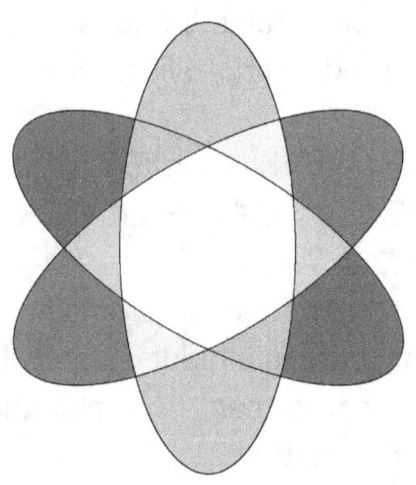

胸腺の活性化を体感した話
A story about experiencing the activation of the thymus

　上昇気流（アセンション）体験や覚醒体験を経て思うことがあります。
　There are things I think about after experiencing an ascending current (ascension) experience and an awakening experience.

　アセンションのクライマックスあたりに起こる現象の一つに胸腺（きょうせん）の活性化があります。肌感覚で体感できるレベルで胸腺の活性化が起こります。
　One of the phenomena that occurs around the climax of ascension is the activation of the thymus. Activation of the thymus occurs at a level that can be felt through the skin.

　その時の現象を文字にすると、熱く滾（たぎ）る胸の中心と言いますか、心臓の少し上あたりに蝶（ちょう）のような蝶番（ちょうつがい）のようなイメージのエネルギー体を感じました。そのことを翼（つばさ）と表現しても良いかもれません。熱く滾（たぎ）る日の鳥と表現しても過言ではないかもしれません。

If I were to put the phenomenon at that time into words, I would say that I felt an energy body in the center of my heart, a little above my heart, like a hinge like a butterfly. You might call it wings. It may not be an exaggeration to describe it as a bird of a burning hot sun.

　その胸腺の感覚を感じた時に、小４と言う言葉が連想されました。その頃の感覚を思い出して、あの頃の感覚って一番正しかった気がするなぁ。そして、一番良かった気がするなぁ。と思い返すのでした。男女の別がそれほど大きくなかった頃の感覚です…みんなが友達だった頃の感覚です。

　When I felt the sensation of the thymus, I was associated with the word "small 4". I remember the feeling I had when I was in 4th grade, and I think that feeling back then was the most correct. And I think it's the best. I remembered. It feels like when the gender distinction wasn't so big... when everyone was friends.

胸腺が一生涯のうちで一番活性化される時期は小学４年生頃をピークにするのだそうです。小４をピークに胸腺は生涯をかけて７０歳くらいまで萎縮し続けていくそうです。小４と連想された体験と一致していてビックリしました。小４を年齢に換算すると１０歳です。
It seems that the time when the thymus is most activated in one's lifetime peaks around the fourth grade of elementary school. It is said that the thymus will continue to atrophy for the rest of one's life, with a peak in the 4th grade of elementary school, until the age of 70. I was surprised that it matched the experience associated with "4th grade". If you convert "4th grade" into age, it is 10 years old.

【参考文献】wikipedia調べ　https://ja.wikipedia.org/wiki/%E8%83%B8%E8%85%BA

　そう言われてみれば、あの頃を過ぎたあたりくらいから、男女の差が肉体的にも精神的にも大きく現れてきて、気が付いたら、大きな別が生まれていたなぁ。と…
Come to think of it, the difference between men and women began to appear after that time, and before I knew it, there was a big difference between me physically and mentally.

　そんなことあったなぁ…と、思いを巡らすのでした。
I remember that something like that happened a long time ago.

あの頃って、怪我（けが）をしても治りが良かった記憶があります。あれは、胸腺のおかげだったんだぁ。と思い返すのでした。
I remember that even if I got injured at that time, it healed well. I realized again that the healing power at that time was thanks to the thymus.

また、上昇気流（アセンション）体験や覚醒体験をして、胸腺が活性化されてまいりますと、まるで、子供の心を取り戻したかのような感覚を味わえます。
In addition, when the thymus is activated by the ascending air current (ascension) experience and the awakening experience, you can feel as if you have regained the mind of a child.

子供の頃の感覚をリアルに味わえるような感覚です。
It's a feeling that you can really taste the feeling of childhood.

純真な心と言いますか、なんでも楽しむ感覚と言いますか、いつも愉快（ゆかい）で楽しんでいるような、いつも笑っているような、ひじょうに良い、豊（ゆた）かな感覚を味わえます。
You can say it's an innocent heart, or you can say it's a sense of enjoying everything, it's a very good and rich feeling that you're always happy and enjoying yourself and always smiling.

現代の社会に不満を抱いていて、報われていない感覚や、救われていない感覚を、お持ちの方がいらっしゃいましたら、ぜひ、一度、この感覚を味わってみてはいかがでしょうか。

If you are dissatisfied with modern society and have a sense of being unrewarded or unsaved, why don't you experience this feeling once?

　その感覚を味わえるようになってまいりますと、ものの見方や考え方が一新されていって、満足して生きていける。そんな人生に変換していただけたら幸いです。

When you come to be able to enjoy that feeling, your perspective and way of thinking will be renewed, and you will be able to live with satisfaction. I would appreciate it if you could convert it to such a life.

血液検査の結果から見る、表の事情と裏の事情
Blood test results. facts on the surface, facts on the back

　喜びの束（つか）の間、血液検査で見えてきた数値をピックアップします。血液検査の過去データ
　For a moment of joy, I will pick up the numbers that have been seen in the blood test. Historical blood test data.

採取日付 採取時間 伝票名	2016/05/10	2022/02/16	2022/03/09	2022/05/18
		検体検査	検体検査	検体検査
WBC	6120	5240	5450	6780
RBC	563	550	565	552
Hgb	16.0	16.3	16.6	15.5
Hct	47.0	49.0	49.7	46.8
MCV	83	89	88	85
MCH	28.4	29.6	29.4	28.1 L
MCHC	34.0	33.3	33.4	33.1
PLT	24.9	31.9	34.7	37.9
白血球像				
Baso	0.3	0.6	0.7	0.6
Eosino	7.7 H	4.4	8.4 H	3.4
Stab				
Seg				
Neutro	62.3	53.4	46.0	62.7
Lympho	18.8	35.7	39.6	26.7
Mono	10.9 H	5.9	5.3	6.6
その他1	0.0	0.0	0.0	0.0
その他2	0.0	0.0	0.0	0.0
EBL	0.0	0.0	0.0	0.0
リンパ球（実数）	1150.0 L	1870.0 L	2160.0	1810.0 L
好中球（実数）	3810.0	2800.0	2500.0	4250.0
LD/IFCC		148	142	153
CK	83	436 H	90	166
BUN	15.3	11.6	11.9	18.0
CRE	0.91	0.93	0.91	0.84
UA		6.7	5.8	6.0
Na	142	142	142	142
K	3.9	3.9	3.7	3.7
Cl	102	106	105	104
HDL-C		43	40	38 L
LDL-C		172 H	195 H	197 H

２０２２年２月１６日、この日が初めて健康診断で再受診を促され掛かりつけの病院で受信した日です。この日に心臓のエコー検査などを受けて異常なしの診断を受けました。この時に、LDL-C、いわゆるLDLコレステロールの値が高いから、下げる努力をしていきましょうと告げられた日となります。

　February 16, 2022 is the day when I was asked to undergo a medical checkup again for the first time and received it at my family hospital. On this day, he underwent an echocardiogram of the heart and was diagnosed as having no abnormalities. At this time, I was told that my LDL-C, so-called LDL cholesterol, was high and that I should try to lower it.

２０２２年３月９日、この日が、１回目の経過観察日です。数値が悪化しているのがわかります。この当時、それまで毎日の日課だった晩酌を１ヶ月絶ったんだから大丈夫と、まぁまぁ軽い認識をしておりました。が、しかし、結果が出て、考え方を改める方向へと促されていきます。そして、栄養士の方からのアドバイスもあり、適度な運動、ウォーキングをする習慣を身につけていき、食事療法も取り入れていきました。

　March 9, 2022, this day is the 1th transitional observation day. You can see the numbers getting worse. At that time, I thought it would be okay because I stopped drinking drinks, which had been my daily routine, for a month. However, the results are coming out, and I'm going to be urged to change my mindset. Then, with advice from a dietician, I developed a habit of moderate exercise (walking) and adopted diet therapy.

２０２２年５月１８日、この日が、２回目の経過観察日です。個人的には自信がありましたが、しかし、結果は脆くも更なる悪化が認められ、なんでだ？なんでだ？あれだけやったのにって思うような結果でした。この当時、血液検査の結果は悪化しておりますが、体重が激減していたこともあって、主治医の先生から、努力の跡が見られるので薬は処方せず経過観察をして見ましょうと言われ、３ヶ月後に診て見ましょうと言う話でこの日は終わりました。

　May 18, 2022, this day is the second transitional observation day. Personally, I was confident, but the results were even worse, why? Why? It was a result that I thought even though I did that much. However, blood test results were worse, but there was a fact that the weight was drastically reduced. The doctor in charge told me to observe the progress without prescribing medicine because I could see the traces of my efforts. And the day ended with the story that I will see the doctor again in 3 months.

また、栄養士さんからのアドバイスで、袋とじインスタントラーメンの調理法で、それまでは、スープと具材（キャベツなど）と一緒に麺を茹でて、そのまま召し上がっていましたが、麺をスープとは別で茹でて湯切りしていただく方法を提案され、試して見たところ、あのこってりなラーメンが、あっさりラーメンへと変貌する調理法を教えていただいて、これならイケると、俄然やる気になっていたのを思い出します。

　I also got advice from a nutritionist. This is a cooking method to make "Instant noodles in a bag". Until then, the soup, ingredients (cabbage, etc.) and noodles were boiled together and eaten as is. However, the proposed method was to boil the noodles and soup separately, and then drain the noodles. Then, he taught me a cooking method that turns that rich ramen into a light ramen, and I remember suddenly being motivated to do it.

また、運動のウォーキングも、運動公園にある野球場の周りをグルグル回る方法から、景色を観察しながら歩くウォーキング、例えるならば、図書館まで歩いていって、図書館でクールダウンしながら読書して、良い感じになってきたらウォーキングを再開して家に帰るという方法を工夫しながら始めました。

Also, I changed my walking method from walking around the baseball field in the sports park to walking while observing the scenery. For example, I made a route to walk to the library, cool down at the library, read while I was in the mood, resume walking when I felt better, and go home.

　同じ場所をグルグル回るウォーキングは目的がないから飽きてしまいますが、本を読みたいと目的を作って、動機付けて歩くウォーキングであれば意外と楽しめることに気がついたのでした。

Walking in circles around the same place is boring because it has no purpose, but I realized that walking with a motivation to read a book can be surprisingly enjoyable.

　その中でも、半分歩けたらパイナップルジュースを飲んで良しとか、色々なご褒美を自分に与えたり、やり方を工夫していきました。

Among them, I gave myself various rewards, such as drinking pineapple juice when I could walk halfway, and devised ways to do it.

２０２２年８月１０日
August 10, 2022

　そして、満を持して迎えた２０２２年８月１０日。結果が出ました。LDLコレステロールと書かれている場所を観察していただければ、LDLコレステロールの値が下がっていっているのがわかるかと思います。

　And then, on August 10, 2022, the long-awaited day came. I got results. If you observe the place where LDL cholesterol is written, you will see that the value of LDL cholesterol is decreasing.

No	検査項目	結果	下限値	上限値	コメント	コメント2	単位名称
1	白血球数	5590	3500	9700			/MCL
2	赤血球数	533	M438	577			マン/MCL
3	血色素量	15.0	M13.6	18.3			G/DL
4	ヘマトクリット	46.2	M40.4	51.9			%
5	MCV	87	M 83	101			FL
6	MCH	28.1 L	M28.2	34.7			PG
7	MCHC	32.5	M31.8	36.4			%
8	血小板数	29.9	14.0	37.9			マン/MCL
9	白血球像						
10	好塩基球	0.5	0.0	2.0			%
11	好酸球	5.0	0.0	7.0			%
12	桿状核球		0.0	19.0			%
13	分葉核球		27.0	72.0			%
14	好中球	45.2	42.0	74.0			%
15	リンパ球	42.9	18.0	50.0			%
16	単球	6.4	1.0	8.0			%
17	その他1	0.0		0.0			%
18	その他2	0.0		0.0			%
19	赤芽球	0.0		0.0			/100WBC
20	リンパ球（実数）	2400.0		GT 2000			/MCL
21	好中球（実数）	2520.0					/MCL
22	LD/IFCC	136	120	245			U/L
23	CK	109	M 50	230			U/L
24	尿素窒素	14.6	8.0	20.0			MG/DL
25	クレアチニン	0.93	M 0.65	1.09			MG/DL
26	尿酸	6.7	M 3.6	7.0			MG/DL
27	ナトリウム	142	135	145			MEQ/L
28	カリウム	4.1	3.5	5.0			MEQ/L
29	クロール	108	98	108			MEQ/L
30	総コレステロール	212	150	219			MG/DL
31	中性脂肪	206 H	50	149			MG/DL
32	HDLコレステロール	40	M 40	80			MG/DL
33	LDLコレステロール	155 H	70	139			MG/DL

しかし、注意点があります。栄養士さんからのご指摘がありました。ウォーキングの時どんなドリンクを飲まれていますか？と問われたので、即答でパイナップルジュースです。って答えました。すると、栄養士さんの方が合点がいかれたようで「それだ」って言われました。僕は目が飛び出るように驚きました。笑。
　However, there is a caveat. I was advised by a nutritionist. What kind of drink do you drink when you walk? I was asked, so I immediately answered that it was pineapple juice. Then, the nutritionist seemed to get the point and said "That's it". I was so surprised that my eyes popped out. smile.

　どうやら、甘いドリンクを飲むと中性脂肪が高くなるんだそうです。そこで、ウォーキングの際は、完全にパイナップルジュースを辞めるのは大変だろうから、お茶や麦茶などと交互に飲んでくださいねって愛嬌（あいきょう）の意をいただきました。
　Apparently, when you drink sweet drinks, it seems that " neutral fat " will be high. Therefore, when walking, it would be difficult to completely quit pineapple juice, so he told me to alternate drinking with green tea or barley tea.

と、目に見えるお話はここまでとして、ここからは、思いっきり常識を吹っ飛ばしたようなお話をしてまいります。
　With that said, I will leave the visible story to this point, and from here on I will talk about things that blow away common sense. It's an invisible story.

　２０１９年７月１０日より、クリスタルヒーリングを伝授され、毎日のようにように執り行っていった結果、半年後にアセンションを体験しました。それ以来、毎日のようにアセンションさせる日々を過ごしていき、２０２２年５月中旬頃、恐怖体験を伴（ともな）う覚醒体験をしました。覚醒体験へと移り進む過程にて、たまたま血液検査をしていたわけでした。
　From July 10, 2019, I was taught crystal healing, and as a result of performing it almost every day, I experienced ascension half a year later. Since then, I have spent my days ascending almost every day, and around mid-May 2022, I had an awakening experience accompanied by a frightening experience. In the process of moving to the awakening experience, I happened to have a blood test.

　では、２０２２年５月１８日の資料を見てまいりましょう。
　Let's take a look at the materials for May 18, 2022.

２０２２年５月１８日、血液検査の結果
Blood test results on May 18, 2022

No	検査項目	結果		下限値	上限値	コメント	コメント2	単位名称
1	白血球数	6780		3500	9700			/MCL
2	赤血球数	552		M438	577			マン/MCL
3	血色素量	15.5		M13.6	18.3			G/DL
4	ヘマトクリット	46.8		M40.4	51.9			%
5	MCV	85		M 83	101			FL
6	MCH	28.1	L	M28.2	34.7			PG
7	MCHC	33.1		M31.8	36.4			%
8	血小板数	37.9		14.0	37.9			マン/MCL
9	白血球像							
10	好塩基球	0.6		0.0	2.0			%
11	好酸球	3.4		0.0	7.0			%
12	桿状核球			0.0	19.0			%
13	分葉核球			27.0	72.0			%
14	好中球	62.7		42.0	74.0			%
15	リンパ球	26.7		18.0	50.0			%
16	単球	6.6		1.0	8.0			%
17	その他1	0.0			0.0			%
18	その他2	0.0			0.0			%
19	赤芽球	0.0			0.0			/100WBC
20	リンパ球（実数）	1810.0	L		GT 2000			/MCL
21	好中球（実数）	4250.0						/MCL
22	LD/IFCC	153		120	245			U/L
23	CK	166		M 50	230			U/L
24	尿素窒素	18.0		8.0	20.0			MG/DL
25	クレアチニン	0.84		M 0.65	1.09			MG/DL
26	尿酸	6.0		M 3.6	7.0			MG/DL
27	ナトリウム	142		135	145			MEQ/L
28	カリウム	3.7		3.5	5.0			MEQ/L
29	クロール	104		98	108			MEQ/L
30	総コレステロール	241	H	150	219			MG/DL
31	中性脂肪	125		50	149			MG/DL
32	HDLコレステロール	38	L	M 40	80			MG/DL
33	LDLコレステロール	197	H	70	139			MG/DL

この当時は、まだ、覚醒体験はしておりません。が、しかし、覚醒体験へと移り進む過程であったことは間違いありません。いわゆる、恐怖体験真（ま）っ只中（ただなか）の頃だったと思い返します。正確には２０２２年５月２７日に堪（たま）り兼（か）ねて病院に縋（すが）っていっていますし、２０２２年５月２１日の頃には当時ネット販売していた天然石ショップを閉じる決断をした閉店クーポンを発行している形跡があるので、おそらく、時期的に、かごめの話などが現れていた頃だと推測しています。

　At this time, I have not yet had an awakening experience. However, there is no doubt that it was a process of transitioning to an awakening experience. I recall that I was in the midst of a so-called fearful experience. To be precise, on May 27, 2022, I am stuck at the hospital. Around May 21, 2022, there is evidence that a closing coupon was issued that decided to close the natural stone shop that was selling online at that time, so it was probably around the time when Kagome's story appeared.

　その当時の血液の資料があるなんて、奇跡としか言いようがありません。よくぞ受診して血液検査していたなぁ。と今となっては健康診断に感謝しています。
　I can only say that it is a miracle that there is a blood document from that time. I think I had a blood test at a good timing. And now I am grateful for the health checkup.

実際問題、覚醒体験をいつしたのかと言われると、正直、いつ、覚醒体験をしたのかは定かではありません。２０２２年６月初旬頃だったんだろうなと今、思い返します。

In fact, when asked when I had my awakening experience, I honestly don't know when I had my awakening experience. I think it was around the beginning of June 2022.

なぜ、この貴重な体験が曖昧（あいまい）になっているのかと言うと、覚醒体験へ移り進んで行く最中（さいちゅう）は、本当に何もかもを手放して行く過程にありました。２００万円かけて始めた天然石屋も閉店させ、それまで出版してきた本を全部廃盤にしたり、それまで発信してきた note のアカウントを完全に削除したりと、まぁ、まぁ、記録が残っていないのです。断片を洗いざらいして、だいたいこの辺にこんなことがあったよね。といった具合で、その当時の必死さを思い返します。

The reason why this precious experience has become ambiguous is that in the process of moving on to the awakening experience, I was really in the process of letting go of everything. He also closed the Tennen Ishiya, which he had started at a cost of 2 million yen, discontinued all the books he had published up to that point, and completely deleted the accounts he had posted up to that point. And, well, well, there are no records left.

実際問題、当時は、本当に、それどころではなかった。
In fact, at the time, I couldn't do anything.

なぜならば、ヒーリングを人に伝えることにすら抵抗を覚えていたからです。こんな苦しい思いをするんだったら教えない方が良いのではないか、そもそも、アセンションや覚醒体験を望んでいる人がいるとも限らないし、僕のただの自己満足なんだったら、伝えることをやめた方がいいのではないかとか考えていました。

Because I was reluctant to even tell people about healing. If healing causes such pain, it would be better not to teach it. In the first place, it is not necessarily the case that there are people who want ascension and awakening experiences. I was thinking that if it was just my self-satisfaction, I should stop telling them.

しかし、その体験後、正常に戻っていく体と、健常になる心と、思いがけない発見。覚醒体験へと移り進む過程にて発生する胸腺（きょうせん）の感覚。もしかしたら、この胸腺（きょうせん）の感覚を用いたヒーリングを伝授すれば、世の中の誰かが救われるかもしれないと思うようになってくると、ヒーリングを伝えて行く原動力になっていきました。

However, after that experience, my body returned to normal, my mind became healthy, and I made an unexpected discovery. A thymic sensation that occurs in the process of transitioning to an awakening experience. When I started to think that maybe someone in the world could be saved if I taught healing using this thymus sense, it became the driving force to teach healing.

　胸腺は人間の免疫機能の中枢、中核を担う存在で、コロナやガンから身を守るＴ細胞（Ｔリンパ球）を成熟させる器官であることがわかってきます。胸腺を活性化さすることさえできれば、人間の免疫機能を強化向上させることができると言えるのではないかと素人ながらに思えてならないわけであります。

The thymus plays a central role in human immune function, and it is now known that it is an organ that matures T cells (T lymphocytes) that protect the body from corona and cancer. Even though I am an amateur, I can't help thinking that if we can activate the thymus, we can say that we can strengthen and improve the human immune function.

そう言ったことが見えてきて、初めて、胸腺活性化ヒーリングを公開するに至った訳でありました。
　It was only after I realized this that I was able to open the Thymus Activation Healing to the public.

また、２０２２年７月１９日に、家庭内にコロナ陽性患者が出て保健所の指示に従い一週間程、隔離生活をしました。
　Also, on July 19, 2022, there was a corona-positive patient at home, and I was quarantined for about a week according to the instructions of the public health center.

　その際に胸腺活性化ヒーリングをして、どうなるのか様子をみてみたところ、僕自身、喉（のど）がイガイガするくらいの症状は出たものの、咳（せき）や発熱などの症状は出ることがなく、一週間の隔離生活を無事に過ごすことができました。
　At that time, I did thymus activation healing and saw what would happen. When I tried it, I myself had symptoms that made my throat irritated, but I didn't have any symptoms such as coughing or fever, and I was able to spend a week of quarantine safely.

　たまたま、僕にコロナが移らなかっただけか、胸腺活性化ヒーリングのおかげなのかはわかりませんが、難を逃れることができました。
　I don't know if it just happened that I didn't get the coronavirus or because of the thymus activation healing, but I was able to escape the difficulty.

また、コロナ陽性患者の方にも、胸腺活性化ヒーリングを伝授して、経過観察をしてみたところ、重症化せずに済んでいます。もちろん、薬のお陰もあってのことだとは思いますが、コロナ陽性患者の方が言うには、胸腺活性化ヒーリングを行うことによって気分的に楽になったと事後報告を受けています。

　In addition, when I taught the thymus activation healing to the corona-positive patients and observed their progress, they did not become severe. Of course, I think it was because of the medicine, but I have received reports from corona-positive patients that they felt better after performing thymus activation healing.

　ちなみにですが、うちの家族は全員、稀に見る、ワクチン未接種者です。そんな環境でも軽症で済んでいます。

　By the way, my family is all rare unvaccinated people. Even in such an environment, there are no serious corona patients.

この経験後、２０２２年８月１０日に通院して血液検査を受けてきました。
After this experience, I went to the hospital on August 10, 2022 and received a blood test.

覚醒体験へと移り進む過程で奇跡的に血液検査をした結果と、覚醒体験を経てコロナにも打ち勝った後に血液検査をした結果を見比べてみると面白い結果が見えてきます。
If you compare the results of a blood test miraculously performed in the process of moving to the Awakening Experience and the results of a blood test after overcoming the corona after going through the Awakening Experience, you will see interesting results.

２０２２年５月１８日（覚醒体験前）
　リンパ球数（実数）　1810.0 /MCL
　好中球（実数）4250.0 /MCL
May 18, 2022 (Before Awakening Experience)
Lymphocyte count (real number) 1810.0/MCL
Neutrophils (real number) 4250.0/MCL

２０２２年８月１０日（覚醒体験後）
　リンパ球数（実数）　2400.0 /MCL
　好中球（実数）2520.0 /MCL
August 10, 2022 (after the awakening experience)
Lymphocyte count (real number) 2400.0/MCL
Neutrophils (real number) 2520.0/MCL

もちろん、５月は花粉やカビが増殖する期間であることなど考察すると、季節的な数値の変化もあるでしょうし、一概にリンパ球数が上がっていれば良いと言う訳でもなくて、バランスが取れていることが求められています。
　Of course, considering that pollen and mold grow in May, there will be seasonal changes in the numbers. It does not necessarily mean that it is good if the lymphocyte count is rising, but it is required that it is in balance.

　なぜならば、リンパ球数が異常に高くなると、それはそれで病気と疑われますし、リンパ球数が異常に低くなると、それはそれで病気を疑われます。
　This is because when the lymphocyte count is abnormally high, it is suspected as a disease, and when the lymphocyte count is abnormally low, it is suspected as a disease.

　ですので、一概に量が多ければ良いと言うことではなくて、バランスが取れていて、尚且つ、活性化されていることが肝となります。
　Therefore, it is not necessarily the case that the larger the quantity, the better. The key is to be balanced, yet activated.

　ですので、この数値から胸腺が活性化されたと判定することはできないと自覚しますが。結果的に数値は良いなぁって思っています。今、俺、健全だ。

Therefore, I am aware that it is not possible to judge that the thymus is activated from this value. I think the numbers are good as a result. I'm healthy now.

また、胸腺活性化ヒーリングで胸腺が活性化されたと評価する方法が見つかっていない現状に気が付いています。どうすれば、胸腺が活性化されたと評価できるのか知りたいなぁと思い始めています。

Also, I am aware of the current situation that no method has been found to evaluate that the thymus has been activated by thymus activation healing. I would like to know how to evaluate that the thymus is activated.

答えは見えているんだけど、どうやれば実証できるのかが謎なんです。

I can see the answer, but how to prove it is a mystery.

これからの課題だと自認しております。

I am convinced that this will be an issue for the future.

おわりに AT THE END

　本編にある愛と友情を用いたエネルギーの使い方を実践していきますと、3ヶ月後から半年後あたりで、ハートに昇る龍となる、上昇気流（アセンション）が起こるようになります。
　If you practice how to use energy using love and friendship in the main story, after about 3 to 6 months, an ascending current (ascension) will occur that will become a dragon rising to your heart.

　初めて起きた時、驚きました。そして、愛と友情のエネルギーを用いることの素晴らしさに気づくようになります。
　When the first ascension occurred, I was amazed. You will come to realize how wonderful it is to use the energy of love and friendship.

　上昇気流（アセンション）は実際に起こるものだと、実在する話だと信じるようになりました。
　I came to believe that the ascension was a real thing, a real story.

そして、上昇気流（アセンション）を続けて行った結果、ハートから喉奥（のどおく）へと上昇気流（アセンション）が移り進んで行きます。

And as a result of continuing the ascending current, the ascending current moves from the heart to the back of the throat.

さらに、上昇気流（アセンション）を進めていきますと、頭蓋（ずがい）の中へと移り進んで行きます。しかし、ここまでは、純粋な快楽です。心地の良いものですし、幸せを享受（きょうじゅ）していました。

Furthermore, as you continue to advance the updraft (ascension), you will move into the skull. But so far, it's pure pleasure. It felt good and I was happy.

しかし、僕の例で言いますと、愛と友情を用いたエネルギーの使い方を実践し始めて２年と１０ヶ月が過ぎた頃、頭蓋（ずがい）の中へと移り進んだ先、頭頂部に上昇気流が移り進んで行く最中（さなか）に、地獄の苦しみが現れ出でました。

However, in my example, after two years and ten months of practicing the use of love and friendship energies, the ascension moved into the skull and then into the crown of the head. In the midst of the shifting updraft, hellish torments emerged.

それまでの快楽とは一変して踠（もが）き苦しみます。寒気や悪寒や恐怖や不安にさいなまれ、苦楽を共にするアセンションへと進化していきました。

It's completely different from the pleasure until then, and I'm going to suffer. I was tormented by chills, fear and anxiety. Then it evolved into an updraft (Ascension) of shared suffering and joy.

　この先に起こる覚醒体験のことは、本書で詳しく説明してあります。是非、本書をループして読み起こして見てください。
　The ensuing awakening experience is described in detail in this book. Please loop this book and read it.

　それでは、最後に、胸腺活性化ヒーリングを伝授します。
　Finally, I will teach you about thymus activation healing.

胸腺（きょうせん）活性化ヒーリング
Thymus activation healing

若き日のあなたにお伝え申します。
I would like to tell you in your youth.

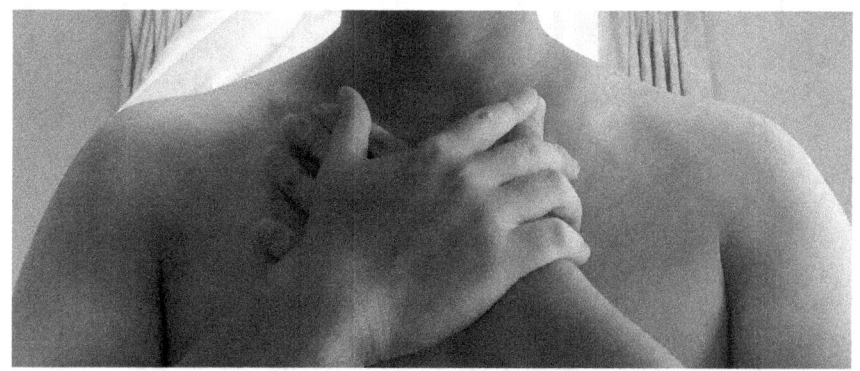

　まず、左手親指を左側の鎖骨に当たるようにセットして、左手人差し指を右側の鎖骨に当たるようにセットしていただきます。そして、右手親指を左手人差し指上あたりに置き、右手人差し指を左手親指上あたりに置いてください。

　First, place your left thumb on your left clavicle and your left index finger on your right clavicle. Place your right thumb above your left index finger and your right index finger above your left thumb.

　正確ではありませんが、だいたいその辺りに胸腺があると想像してください。そもそも、胸腺の位置は覚醒体験へと進む過程で体感していくことなので、ここでは言及を避けておきます。だいたい、あってればOKです。

It's not accurate, but imagine that the thymus is roughly around that area. In the first place, the position of the thymus is to be experienced in the process of advancing to the awakening experience, so I will avoid mentioning it here.

それでは、息をふぅ〜っと吐き出してください。息を吐き出しきったら、素早く息を吸い込み、ゆっくり息を吐き出しながら、胸腺に伝えていきます。
Focus your attention on your breathing.
Say it with your heart as you exhale.

あなた様に愛と友情をささげます。
わたしはあなた様を愛しております。
わたしはあなた様と友達です。
"I dedicate my love and friendship to you."
"I love you."
"I'm friends with you."

声に出さず、心の声でお呟(つぶや)きください。これを息継ぎのたびに繰り返していきます。今のあなたに、時間的余裕があるなら、そのまま瞑想をしましょう。※特に瞑想する時間に決まりはありません。あなたの赴(おもむ)くままに心地よいだけ行っていただけたらと思います。
Don't say it out loud, but mutter in your heart. Repeat with each breath. If you have time now, let's just meditate. *There is no set time to meditate. I would like you to go as comfortable as you want.

ハートの中心より出てまいります、愛と友情のエネルギーの感覚を感じられた方はいらっしゃいますか？または、イメージやビジョン、サウンドやミュージック、動画や物語など、様々な形で何かを見せてくれるかもしれません。

Can anyone feel the energy of love and friendship emanating from the center of their hearts? Alternatively, they may show us something in various forms, such as images and visions, sounds and music, videos and stories.

そんな感覚、感じがきたら、自分でこさえないで、もっと見せてくださいと言うように、抗わずに進んで体験していきましょう。これは自己に内在する存在が動き出しているその証拠なんです。

If you feel that way, don't hold back and go ahead and experience it as if you want to see more of it. This is the proof that the existence inherent in the self is starting to move.

また、愛と友情のエネルギーの使い方をして起きたことは忘れないうちにメモにとっておきましょう。

Also, before you forget what happened when you used the energy of love and friendship, make a note of it.

僕の本はこのメモから作られています。

My book is made from this memo.

www.ingramcontent.com/pod-product-compliance
Lightning Source LLC
Chambersburg PA
CBHW052349220526
45465CB00003BA/1026